CW00520810

PATHWAY INTO SUNRISE

The author

Esmé Ellis is an artist trained at the Royal College of Art. Since wrestling with and recovering from M.E., she has been leading workshops and groups in spiritual and psychological self-awareness, using meditation, art, and healing as the means to inner growth and self-healing. She is now completing a prophetic and visionary work of science fiction.

PATHWAY INTO SUNRISE
Journey of a Wounded Healer

by

ESMÉ ELLIS

Illustrated by Carol Lambert and the author

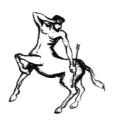

Published by
Horus Books

First published in 1998
by
Horus Books,
P.O. Box 2529, Bath, BA2 6XR

Foreword © Dr Kai Kermani, 1998

The poem 'Descent' by Esmé Ellis was
first published in *Poet's Voice* 1985

The poem 'Untitled' on page 223 is
© Rose Flint, 1997

ISBN 0-9533928-0-5

A catalogue record for this book is available from the
British Library

Copy-editing, design and typesetting by
Mushroom Publishing, Bath, UK

Printed and Bound in Great Britain by
Cox & Wyman, Reading

DEDICATION

To Sandhya
for your inspirational birthday gifts,
the best of which was yourself.

ACKNOWLEDGEMENTS

My heartfelt thanks to the many friends, too many to mention individually, though they will know who they are, who have encouraged and supported me on this venture. My especial gratitude to Michael who has upheld me; to Dr Max Mayer for his generous, warm friendship and faith in me, sustained over almost 40 years; to Martyn Folkes who has made all things possible; and to Rose Flint who has constantly inspired me through difficult times and joyful moments, and who has truly midwifed this book through to birth.

Some names have been changed to avoid identification; others keep their real names.

CONTENTS

FOREWORD

Dr Kai Kermani BSc, MRCS, MRCGP, DRCOG

As a physician and scientist, I used to think that with our progressively advancing technology, medical science, and the pharmaceutical industry, I would have all the answers and the tools to treat effectively all the patients that streamed through my door. However, I have now discovered that in my arrogance and blinkered vision of health and disease, which was instilled in me as part of my medical training, I had actually learnt to ignore and alienate the individual's spiritual dimension and their innate and immense healing powers. I was thus inadvertently and unknowingly dis-empowering them in my attempts to treat them.

I now realise that each individual's life journey is unique, and their healing potential is unlimited. Apart from our still inadequate medical technology and social conditioning, which continues to propagate negative belief systems, the main factor that seems to prevent the full realisation of the healing potential is the individual's unawareness of its existence. Engaging the clients/patients in a truly holistic vision of themselves, their bodies, minds, emotions and spirit, not only enables them to overcome their distress, disease or disability, but empowers them to move forward and discover that inner source of sacred unconditional spiritual love and healing energy.

In this beautifully descriptive book, Esmé Ellis chronicles her own personal journey through life and some of its fears, disease and dark spaces. It offers one person's extraordinary experience of healing and recovery from devastating ME, through the intervention of spiritual energy and the appearance of her teaching guide Astrazzurra. An experience she calls a 'medium-sized miracle'. I strongly and genuinely share with her the belief that the miracle is not necessarily just in the recovery, but in the fact that each and everyone of us has the potential to do exactly the same or more. Although the process would be totally different and unique for each one of us, we all have the innate power and potential to soar up to the skies and rise above our perceived limitations, in order to manifest the truth and reality of this strength and power in our lives with the help of the Divine's gracious unconditional love, light and healing.

I greatly admire the absolute honesty and total courage with which Esmé has exposed her deepest fears, pains, and inner self in recounting her gripping, enthralling, and moving life story. But then it is only by acknowledging our shadow side, and going into the depths of our worst nightmares and emotions, with the help of our spiritual guide, Higher Self or a therapist/healer, that we can lay the ghosts of the past to rest, and move on towards achieving our unlimited full potential and healing.

She managed to achieve this admirably, against the background of a lack of understanding among an unenlightened section of the medical and nursing profession. It was a great honour and a privilege to be a part of her journey in writing this Foreword, as she beautifully demonstrates the triumph of intense desire for self survival. Her story should act as an inspiration to anyone who is travelling through the dark night of the Soul in their journey of life.

Dr. Kermani is a GP and member of most of the Royal Colleges and scientific and holistic medical organisations. He is also a stress management consultant, international lecturer and workshop facilitator, and author of the highly successful book Autogenic Training.

INTRODUCTION

What draws us to a particular path in life? Which of the seemingly random seeds that destiny scatters before us will sprout and perhaps flower, which will shrivel? What urge was it that led me to choose sculpture as a career, and why did I find myself immobilised, paralysed by disease, unable even to hold a pencil just when my chosen career seemed to be on the point of success and my marriage less than two months old? Out of my sense of devastation and grief at the shattering of my life's dreams, despairing questions arose. Why has this happened? I haven't deserved it. Why? Gradually answers began to come and a deeper understanding emerged.

Fascination with the elements – earth and water, fire and air – stirred some unnamed force within me from the earliest age. I was making mud-pies in the backyard almost before I could walk. By the age of seven I'd been initiated by the local children into the strange childhood mystery of fashioning little touch-boxes out of clay dug from the ground. We would bake them in the sun until they hardened. Then, packing one tiny chamber with dry, decaying wood it would be ignited with an ember, blown upon gently, cupped in our hands as it spluttered and threatened to fade before finally smouldering into life. After attaching a thick string, it was ready to launch. We would swing the little clay vessel round our heads in wider and wider circles and it would begin to glow in the autumn twilight, emitting a trail of sparks like a fiery comet. This seems to me to be quite a metaphor! I learned many years later that Henry Moore had also participated in this ancient mystery in his own Yorkshire childhood, and that this instinctive contact with common clay had called out of him, too, an intuitive desire to sculpt. Sculpture, the most ancient of all the arts, links us to the very earth-root of humankind's creativity, as well as to the starry skies.

I was given a place at the local junior art school at the age of eleven, and graduated from the sculpture school of the Royal College of Art thirteen years later determined to make this art form my life's work. Then I was struck down by a severe case of M.E. At this point my life faltered, almost petered out, but then changed completely.

Myalgic encephalomyelitis has had so much publicity in recent years that there must be very few who haven't heard of it. Yet it can vary so widely in the way it is experienced by different people that there can't be a simple description of it. Indeed, it goes by so many names that it is hard to pin down. Post Viral Fatigue Syndrome being one instance, which seems to imply feeling rather run down after 'flu. Yet the fatigue which I and countless other sufferers experienced is quite unlike any ordinary fatigue. Even the deepest exhaustion encountered in normal life fails to convey its effect.

In the late sixties and early seventies there was virtually no recognition of the reality of the illness, and the message I was being given by the medical profession in general, though there were honourable exceptions, was that it was 'all in the mind'. I should pull myself together and find some real work - something other than this airy-fairy sculpture – and I would soon snap out of it. So being half persuaded that they might be right, I took up teaching and pushed myself into such a state of exhaustion that eventually all the systems in my body collapsed. I entered a nightmare of intense pain. I was unable to feed or wash myself or turn over in bed. Worse still I couldn't hold a conversation, read, listen to the radio or TV throughout two long years of living death. My life disintegrated. Everything, it seemed, had been snatched away.

Yet out of this black hole something remarkable emerged. A medium sized miracle. In the darkest, most desperate moment of my life a dazzling blue light appeared, and with it the dawning realisation that I had a spiritual teacher who wanted to communicate. Simultaneously, I became aware of an inner healer who conferred on me the ability to heal my life and the power to heal others.

My relationship with this guide or teacher, who I have called *Astrazzurra*, developed into a supportive, loving friendship. Life took on new dimensions. It became an adventure – a journey of discovery. In sharing it with you, I hope to show how one person's experience, unique and individual as it is, is also universal. I was not singled out from the rest of humanity to receive this amazing illumination and healing. The guidance and support, which came to me from the 'other world', is available to everyone, and will become more readily so in the near future. Only we have to do our part in crossing the bridge that divides the two worlds. We must learn to sense these other realities, becoming consciously open and receptive, yet without losing our sense of responsibility and discernment.

This is a story of inspiration and hope, a journey in which there is the discovery that Healing, Loving and Creativity go hand in hand. That the spiritual healing of disease is not just an episode in life which restores us to the level of health we had before, but can be an unfolding and awakening to our true life's purpose. I shall begin at the beginning where all good stories begin, since it is important that this episode is not taken out of context, but is viewed as part of the journey of life in its wholeness. The new age before us as we cross the threshold, not only of a new century but a new millennium, offers us the opportunity to step into the Light. Into new understanding and new dimensions. I hope you will discover, as I did, the power that transforms and heals your life.

ONE

I am told that the Greeks have a saying
that at the moment of your birth
is born also a worm which
is waiting to meet you.

ROOTS

My birth was, as it could be said of most of us, an event both commonplace and unique. A blizzard had been blowing and there was some anxiety that the midwife would not be able to get through the deep snow which had been falling all night. It was March 1934, the period just after the great depression and a few short years before the Second World War. Somewhere between the twin shadows of these events I made my entrance.

I was the offspring of a kind and hardworking father and a caring, well meaning mother. The birth took place in a bedroom above a small grocer's shop. It overlooked the backyard that we shared with the butcher next door. The scene must have been fairly typical of the poorer, work-a-day fringes of any northern industrial city at that time. Drab and featureless paving stones, soot-darkened brick walls, and windows smeared with whitening, which served as curtains for our neighbour's shop, was the immediate view. A narrow stretch of earth and grass bounded by a tall, overgrown, privet hedge and more brick walls, completed the picture.

My parents had made a brave attempt to make of it a garden – sown grass seeds, put in a few plants – but in that discouraging environment the plants were struggling against the odds. Rather like the people in the neighbourhood around them. My mother took a pride in this, her first home as a married woman, and in the appearance and well being of her first-born and, as it turned out, only child. Fresh air, she knew, was good for babies, so as the snows melted and the warmer days of spring came along, I was wrapped up in hand knitted shawls and woollies and put out in my pram. But our neighbour's side of the tiny backyard was a wasteland. A patch of burnt earth where rubbish had been incinerated, and fringing it, lank grass and rank weeds surrounding a row of battered bins.

It is odd how that earth has impressed itself upon me. I can see myself a year or two later. A fair, curly-headed toddler in a clean romper suit, playing in the garden, digging and scraping about in that impoverished soil with a big spoon and paddling it into mud pies. It was a dead mouse-grey and full of stones.

How far back can one's memory go? I certainly remember being put out in that big, black, deep-bellied pram and I remember its textures and its smell quite clearly. I can't say what it smelled like, because it wasn't a smell *like* anything else. Not even like another pram. Its smell was of *that* pram. I can recall once rocking it from side to side more and more violently until I deliberately tipped it over, knowing it would bring my mother screaming with panic out of her kitchen.

But is it possible, I wonder, to remember much further back? How far can I go back? To the beginning? Was there any awareness at all of those days surrounding my birth? If I scan my mind and try to recapture my earliest impressions, it is as though a part of me was inside the consciousness of a tiny cell in which a primitive sense is awakening. I am trying to discover, in some sensory way, what manner of place I am coming into. I feel like a seed which is being blown in on the wind, and, drawn by an innate desire for earth, it puts out fine tendril-like roots. At the same time, another part of me is outside watching over – looking down from a distance.

My impressions now as I survey the scene are quite detached. I view myself, the tiny being who is about to enter the stage, as one insignificant speck of humanity in a crowd, one pebble among the multitude piled up on a beach. In this state of detachment it seems to me that at any one moment numberless millions of drab lives are being lived, each of them the result of millions more lives going endlessly back into the past. What is there to distinguish any one from the others? Like a ploughed field full of dull stones, why would anyone bend down to select one and examine it? From a distance they are all the same and all as featureless. Of what use or interest can this particular one be to anyone else?

Yet nothing on God's earth is worthless. The very act of looking begins to unlock one secret after another. I move in closer and focus as the sun begins to glint on colour and sparkle. My attention is caught. I am drawn in. Disinterest gradually gives way to interest. Nothing – no thing – exists by chance. Perhaps every one of those plain, unprepossessing pebbles encapsulates a story. And if *one* plain pebble can reveal surprises, surely this must be true of them all. Soon there comes an understanding of a common heritage that unites mankind one with another, and with the source from which we all came. That source which has been called the Divine or the Creator.

I look back at my birthplace again with growing interest. Was this really the place where I began? I know *now* that I wasn't born here by chance, so I will regard the scene a little more closely and with a little more feeling. I will let it open up to me little by little and see what it has to tell me, and perhaps I'll be rewarded. What sort of community is this?

What people are these that I came to make my home with I wonder? Though my first impressions register lives overlaid by an aura of drabness and poverty, it doesn't seem a squalid or abject existence by any means. They seem friendly and cheerful as well as industrious, and if they are hard working it is because they believe it will lead to better things. They see themselves as a new generation with enterprise and determination who, having caught the spirit of the times, are stepping out, despite the pervading economic depression, beyond the limitations of their background.

The generation from which most of these people sprang were self-employed craftsmen and women, labourers on local farms or in the new steel-mills: a community steeped in Victorian self-improvement and staunch Methodism. Living in old family farmhouses or cottages, their parents had earned whatever possessions they had and bought their education dearly by long hours of toil for minimum reward. My own grandparents on my father's side had been smallholders and metal craftsmen. Grandfather was a silver refiner when he married. As for my grandmother, I was often told the story of how she had to get up early in the morning to milk a small herd of cows before going to school. This had helped to earn her the penny a week which paid for her schooling.

The village school and the green fields where cows had grazed were gone by the time I was born, and the picture my father painted for me of his own childhood had the quality of fairy stories. He would wave his arms around and get me to imagine Great Uncle Bill's hayfield and his team of horses – just there, where those ugly new corporation houses now stand. Pastures here! Streams meandering through them alive with little darting fish, lost forever beneath the tarmac of the busy street. I would conjure up the scene in my mind as I did when my mother read me stories.

It was hard for me to imagine that my grandparents had ever been children. Even with the help of faded sepia photographs I marvelled at their strange, heavy, tight-laced clothes. Could they ever have been real children, I wondered? How were they able to run and play games like me, and swing upside down on the rails outside the school gates? And what would they have learned in their village school for the price of that penny earned so early in the morning, long before the time I usually awoke? Certainly they had learned to read and write and do their sums. Maybe they learned of the Kings and Queens of old and their battles for territory and power, but little of their own heritage and their important place within it.

Sheffield's reputation world-wide has been based on its cutlery manufacture which was carried out originally in small workshops by the 'little mesters', as they are called locally. A few of these tiny stone sheds with their forges, bellows and benches were standing deserted in out of the way corners of the village in my childhood, but I knew nothing of their purpose then. Even today you can come across the odd timber-framed cottage squeezed in between a dilapidated Victorian terrace and a poorly built 1920's row of houses and no one seems to notice the incongruity. An ancient cruck barn, a type of building begun in the eleventh century, was used as a park keeper's hut until it simply dropped to pieces. Then it was unceremoniously knocked down and replaced with something more up-to-date. Other towns might have restored such pieces of their history, with pride as well as an eye to their commercial potential, but here no such sentiment reigned.

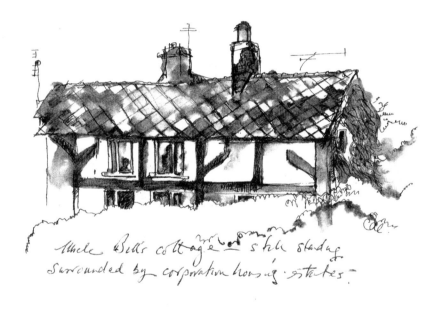

Uncle Bill's cottage still standing
surrounded by corporation housing estates.

The city's name originated in far off times when a family of Angles created a 'feld' or clearing beside the River Sceath and built a settlement there, and Sceath-feld came into being. Two hundred years ago it was still a small town made stinking and grimy by open sewers and the smoking fires of arrow-makers and cutlers. The population grew and the conditions worsened, yet out of the squalor and chaos of its narrow streets a fine degree of craftsmanship emerged. In 1773 an assay office was granted to the city attracting silversmiths eager to make their fortune. The high quality of their craftsmanship coupled with the later inventions of silver plating and stainless steel boosted the city's reputation further. The world famous bowie knives were hand-crafted in cramped workshops down fetid alleyways.

With this fame came a rapid expansion and the city spread outwards, cutting into and eating up the fields and villages as it grew. Very soon, with the coming of mass production, the ear-splitting sounds of rolling mills were shattering the tranquillity of the once peaceful countryside. Heavy steel mills, which now lay all along the Don valley, added to the violation by pouring pollution into the rivers and sulphurous smells into the air from their dark smokestacks and raging furnaces.

As a school child, sometimes taking the long way home on a solitary tram ride or bike ride, I would venture off the safe and beaten track and explore parts of my own city that were beyond my known territory. I felt overawed by the sight of the gigantic steel workshops. I listened to the thunderous earth-shaking rumbles and reverberations issuing from the heavy forges, saw tall chimneys releasing red, purple or ochre clouds, or watched, from a safe distance, the heat of mighty furnaces setting the skies ablaze and aglow in a winter's twilight. I felt fearful and repelled, exhilarated and excited all at the same time.

The old life, a village community living by a mixture of metal craft and farming, was still there when I was born, but it was fast disappearing beneath the sprawl of the city. The repercussions of the Victorian population explosion, which itself had been fuelled by the Industrial Revolution, was rapidly obliterating the cohesion of that rural life with a tide of housing estates and shops. The older generation of grandparents and great aunts, which I knew as a small child, were still baking their bread, tending their fruit and herb gardens, hand-milking their cows and hammering and fettling implements in their small forges. Meanwhile, the brash twentieth century flowed in all around them; a redbrick sea of health centres, cinemas and working men's clubs.

My small world of early childhood was centred in a row of shops each distinguished by their smells and colours. The greengrocers were especially colourful and smellful, with earthy potatoes and fruity reds, greens, oranges and yellows. The fragrant, astringent chemist shop smells, the exciting but difficult-to-put-a-name-to tang of metallic-oily-soapy-woody smells issuing from the hardware shop across the road, intrigued me. Like a small animal I discovered and mapped my world through primitive senses. In the backyard I would trundle Wilfred my toy rabbit and a litter of small dolls around in a tiny pram. Here I became magically enchanted by a cheap Japanese toy: a bird made of paper and a few yellow feathers with cellophane for wings. It was attached to a cane by a string and gave a fluttery whistle as I whirled it around my head. Its fragile translucent wings catching the sun created a rainbow of colour.

This confined area was my place of security. But out front, I was soon to discover, the street was full of sound and movement – the to-ing and fro-ing of people. A young child's consciousness is a series of impressions of happenings and sensations. It doesn't *know*: it experiences. It doesn't know, because knowledge is something built up from experience. So it is those experiences which come along that are its building blocks of knowledge. Early experiences usually make a great impression and condition future behaviour. Like any baby animal or bird, its parents teach, through signals of one sort or another, what is safe and what is dangerous. One of the signals it picks up is the strong approval or disapproval of the grown-up world. Unlike the animal though, the grown-up world also transmits the message BAD versus GOOD. So the child is constantly getting signals, such as 'This is OK' which builds up inside to the feeling, *I am* OK versus *I am* BAD, and IT ISN'T SAFE TO BE BAD. There is a confusion of messages and the young one can't distinguish between the proper concern of its parent for its safety and well being, and some of the admonitions which are aimed at making it conform to the group belief system or social conditioning.

The normal adult's instincts are to bring up their children in a way that is acceptable to the group, and the young child, who is sensitive and pliable, soon gets the idea that compliance is rewarded, and with that it gains a sense of belonging. Looked at in another way this might be called 'brainwashing'. What is the child to do, then, if its experiences are at odds with its parents? Does it try rebellion? Does it test its will? This testing-ground dilemma between child and parent, danger and security, must be as old as humanity itself.

The parent's task in making judgements about where the boundaries can be drawn at each stage of development is as difficult as the child's task in making *its* explorations into life. With each new conception, a new throw of the dice brings together a unique combination of individuals whose attempts to conform or rebel will also be unique. The Cosmos will express itself again and renew itself.

This cosmic view came for me late in life. Yet there were glimmers all along the path. Unfortunately, it took a crisis to bring home the realisation. The experiences which I have undergone in this lifetime, and which have opened up for me the reality of a spiritual dimension, have given me, as it were, an expanded perspective, so that there is now a place where I can begin to view myself from the outside and be a spectator or an observer of events. Detached, while at the same time more under-standing and forgiving. There is a knowledge too that consciousness is not confined within the body, nor within one lifetime that begins at birth and ends at death. Looking back to my beginnings now from the other end of life I can see much that I couldn't see before. I recall an earlier memory still. It is as if I am observing my entry into planet Earth at some moment before my birth. I am looking down from a happy place of sunshine and blue skies and I am joyful and light of being. Something is inexorably pulling me down, and I am reluctant and sad. There is a new sensation, it might be fear. I peep into a little bedroom with flower-sprigged wallpaper. There is a double bed and an alcove with a tiny lace-decorated cot. All empty and quiet and waiting. I can't stay in that room. I am too light. I'm bobbing up again into the sunlight high above, and back into the happy playful laughter.

But I look down once more and see, standing in a patch of sunlight within a small backyard, a grey-haired midwife with a white apron, and she is beckoning me – calling me down. And I am drawn down – grow-ing heavier and needing to breathe the strange air. I forget – Conscious-ness is being wiped clear.

Now, there is no 'before'. Birth is a clean page, a fresh beginning, and the first two or three years can only be recaptured from whatever memo-ries have been impressed with enough force to register on conscious-ness. Something unusually happy or curious or attention grabbing in some way. One or two events begin to stand out from the background of those first three years. The installation of a smart new ice-cream making machine in the shop, and the plying of happy children in summertime with piled cones of vanilla or strawberry home-made ices topped with farm cream. Baskets of brown eggs in straw. A dark November night when fireworks were still being sold after ten or eleven o'clock and I was allowed boxes of green and red Bengal matches to strike, because, unlike ordinary matches, they were thought to be safe in children's hands. Memories of strange salesmen in pinstriped trousers and mono-cles who came to introduce us to new wares, and of being offered tastes of ginger chocolate biscuits or pineapple cheese to try. These tastes stayed with me throughout the years of wartime deprivation that fol-lowed, when the opportunity to indulge tastes of any kind was severely limited.

My memory carries yet another scene. The strong over-sweet scent of masses of privet flowers from the hedge which had never been cut and stood six or seven foot high, mingling with a smell which went to the pit of my stomach and led me, as a toddler, to that row of rusty old dustbins. Open curiosity, despite the smell which intrigued and repelled me at the same time, prompted me to lift the lid and peer into the bin which came up to the height of my nose. I was amazed rather than revolted to discover a seething mass of maggots. Thousands upon thousands, heaving and glistening in endless movement in a shimmer of stinking flesh and bones. I could not move from the spot – it was as if I were hypnotised. Then my mother saw what was happening and flew to snatch me away from the horror. I only have to smell privet flowers now, and… you can imagine the rest.

I don't know which comes first, the learning to talk or the understanding of other people's conversations. Probably the latter, because I certainly remember my mother and father discussing their desire to move and take me to a 'better and healthier place to grow up in'. I had understood their tut-tutting and tones of disapproval and disgust about the conditions at the butcher's shop next door, and knew that they *never* bought meat from their neighbours. We went, instead, to another shop further up the hill. So it was perhaps this constant gossip about the 'awfulness' of next door that made me alert and curious for drama. I was forever peeping out of the window looking for something 'awful', and wasn't disappointed.

The young butcher's boy, a lad of about 12 or 13, since that was the school leaving age then, came out of the back door with a bucket, as he often did. Was I expecting gore and maggots again? I don't know, but he didn't look at all happy. I'd often seen him crying, poor lad. This day he looked unhappy and sick as he began to tip the contents of the bucket down the drain. As they poured out I could see an interesting mess of green and yellowness, and although I couldn't smell it, there must have been an awful stink, for the poor chap fell over on the paving stones in a dead faint. In great glee I ran to my mother crying, 'Look! Look! Come and see!' There was a lot of bother and consternation, and an angry and embarrassed butcher.

This incident proved to be the last straw, particularly since I had such a lot of fun with it. They *must* get me away from all of this as soon as possible and go to live in this 'better' place. Only I had no concept of 'better' because there was no other experience to compare it with, so I was being uprooted from the home I knew and was going into the unknown.

I am discovering that my roots are thirsty and somewhat stunted. Although I received care and love as a baby, the environment I first encountered at birth seemed alien. Where my roots longed for rich, moist, earthy browns and fertile greenness, they found only hard tarmac and dusty earth. Making this journey back to my origins is the beginning of a healing journey. One of the insights that is coming through to me just now is that when healing, in its fullest sense, takes place, then we heal our past as well as our present and our future. Healing, which means 'becoming whole', involves not just the physical body, nor even the emotions, mind and psyche, but it includes the very ground one has trodden. The pavements, buildings, public spaces and interiors one has entered are all woven into us. The squalid and the sordid, the magnificent and the holy are part of our being. Out of this we create, for good or ill, our reality, and participate in the creation of the common reality of humanity.

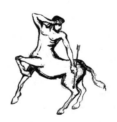

MOVEMENTS, INTERLUDES
AND PRELUDES

The new house was half a mile away up the hill, where there was space and sky. It was again a shared yard but with two distinct gardens divided by a mutual path, and both plots were cultivated and bright with flowers. The garden gate opened into a half-wild field. Our new neighbours were friendly and warmly welcoming, and a recently built school nearby seemed to be just waiting for the day when I would be old enough to go. I was entered for the autumn term and couldn't wait. But first we would take a late summer holiday. It was late August 1939, and we went as a family party with our Leicester aunts, uncles and cousins to Hayling Island somewhere down off the South Coast, a long journey for our little black Ford. The weather was idyllic, and the boarding house had a huge lawn with palm trees and cedars. I was in my seventh heaven. Yet, as we played on the beach and splashed in the sea, all the time a strange sense of foreboding communicated itself to me. I was noticing the strange silences, and the solemn looks on the faces of the grown-ups as they sat side by side on the beach. Out at sea on the horizon large ships were passing, and every so often they would engage in bursts of gunfire. They were so tiny, these ships in the distance, that they looked like toys. We children happily dug sand-scapes on the beach. We filled our buckets from the sea and poured it into the hollows. We made little boats of driftwood and shrieked as we made them go bang and boom at one another. But the grown-ups were snappy with our chatter.

One day in the second week of our holiday we didn't go to the beach at all, but stayed at the house and played in the garden. Then gradually everyone grew solemn and went indoors to listen to the radio, leaving me, as I was the youngest, to amuse myself outside. To begin with I was happy enough. It was a lovely day, and there were clouds of multi-coloured butterflies to chase. But this innocent happiness was soon to be disturbed more deeply and thoroughly than anyone perhaps realised at the time. They eventually came out from the dim sitting-room into the light of the garden with ashen faces. My eldest cousin was crying. Chamberlain had announced to the nation that from 11 a.m. we would be at war with Germany. The next day we packed up and went home, and this time *I* was crying for the loss of my seaside holiday. It was a long time before there were such holidays again.

* * *

I have met several people in recent years, and read books by others, who were born with psychic gifts. People who from an early age were able to 'see' or 'hear' presences or beings from another dimension – a subtler dimension than our physical world. Some of these, as gifted children, were lucky enough to have been born to parents who were themselves psychically and spiritually gifted. Others not so fortunate had to deny and repress the evidence of their sensitive eyes and ears, because their parents and the world in general ridiculed them or totally disbelieved them. I was, for instance, given an account of a sensitive adolescent who had this gift and regularly saw beautiful ethereal figures who seemed to want to make contact and talk with her. She was made so confused and insecure by the rejection of her vision by her parents and those around her, that it affected her physical vision and she began to lose her eyesight. The denial of her own inner vision and truth, and her need to be loved and accepted by those around her, caused the physical body to develop blindness in desperation. I wasn't blessed or cursed with this early psychic sight. And yet... There may have been one or two strange experiences, and I think this may be quite *normal*. Most people will have had the odd experience which couldn't be explained. One such early experience of my own around the age of four was of seeing a fairy!

It was so unremarkable for me at the time that I just said, 'Look, there's a fairy,' just as I might have commented on a butterfly or a wasp. I'd heard about fairies, seen pictures of them with their pink and blue dresses and their gauzy wings and star-topped wands. But this day I was sitting on my mother's knee at the breakfast table, the sun shining through the window and onto my plate. I had a half eaten teacake on my plate. My mother, in a happy mood, was entertaining me with some song or nursery rhyme, when a sudden movement caught my attention, and a tiny insect-like creature alighted on my teacake. I was fascinated and puzzled by it. It was the colour of the piece of food on which it stood, a sort of creamy fawn, and I looked more closely expecting it to be a little moth. But no: it stood upright with a pair of arms down by its side culminating, not so much in fingers, but in flexible wispy 'feelers' such as you might see on the tips of some insect's antennae. I must have watched it closely, because I noticed that it didn't have wings. At least, not the sort of wings that insects have or those fairies I had seen in picture books. As if to answer my curious thoughts about the matter, it raised its tiny arms, and I saw that the fawn coloured dress it was wearing was fluted in tight folds and that its arms were in some way attached to these folds, so that when it raised them above its head they fanned out and became the wing-like means to flight. Most fascinating of all was its curious face. Curious in both senses, as it was not at all pretty, nor was it quite human, yet it looked at me just as I was looking at it, with a rather suspicious but intense interest. I couldn't contain my pleasure any longer and gasped , 'Look, look mother! A fairy'. With which it disappeared. It did not fly away, it disappeared. My memory of the whole thing is clear and precise.

My mother, of course, didn't see anything and told me I was making up stories – fairy stories, I suppose! And as I never saw anything like it again, I let it fade away and learned not to mention it. It was only when, many long years later, I met a very sober and intelligent woman who regularly saw fairies, and whose drawings depicted them as similar in character to the one I had seen in childhood, that I had to rethink my scepticism.

The other important incident from that pre-school year was the appearance of a snake. On washday we had these big heavy clothes-posts that were slotted into post-holes, four or five inches square in the ground, which were removed again when not in use. It had just been raining and when the sun came out I went off to play in the garden. I stopped to look down into the post-hole to see if there was anything of interest, and there, coiled up, was a snake. I crouched down to see him more clearly. He had bright black eyes and shiny skin, and as I observed him more closely I could see a zigzag pattern on his back. His dark eyes were looking at me, but not in the same way that the fairy had done, since there was no sense of meeting and communicating. A shaft of sunlight touched him and I saw tiny diamond-shaped scales on his back reflecting beautiful colours. Deep blues, greens, purples and reds. Maybe it was the effect of the sunlight reflecting off his damp scales, but I wanted to touch my beautiful jewelled snake.

Something held me back, and I thought I'd better go and report my find to the grown-ups. So I ran in to Mrs Jones our neighbour. For some reason her husband was away from work that day, and so I broke my news to both of them. Once again, there was disbelief and also a bit of a hullabaloo as I insisted shrilly, over and over, that there *was* a snake. By this time my mother had heard the commotion and come running over, and eventually they all trooped into the garden. The snake was still there, and this time it began hissing and rearing. Who would blame it, finding itself surrounded by these excited and hysterical adults? At this point, Mr Jones began shepherding them all back indoors and away from danger.

Once inside again, no one seemed to know what to do. Then inspiration struck Mr Jones. He ran into the kitchen and grabbed a jar of salt and a spoon. 'I'll put salt on its tail, that'll shift it,' he cried with triumph, and charged into the garden. This was not the fate I had wanted for my snake, but at least everyone seemed to be taking it seriously. Luckily, by the time he got to the post-hole, the snake had gone. I expect it had made its way to the field beyond the garden. Surprisingly, that seemed to satisfy everyone. It had gone, and that was that.

The snake was real enough but the fairy was quite another matter. The rational explanation for what I saw, the sort of thing that is heard in serious discussions by educated people, our experts on psychology and professional sceptics, is that these are illusions of the mind projected onto some outward object or situation. In order to be projected, there has to be an inner image from which that projection arises. The rational explanation continues: that inner image comes from something we have seen or heard and has perhaps been put away in our unconscious mind and forgotten. But the creature I saw at the age of four had no resemblance to anything I had seen or heard about. It was in no way a pretty, sugary pink, miniature child with butterfly wings, such as all the stories and pictures had led me to believe. I was not looking at something I knew already, but something quite original, which I could not have invented.

* * *

This period of childhood was pleasant and carefree enough, and I had no qualms about the prospect of growing up and becoming big enough to start my first term at school. But the premature homecoming after our holiday in the South threw everyone's plans into chaos. The shop had been left in the hands of a couple of assistants while we were away, and in those few days there had been a spate of panic buying and the shelves were all but empty. I remember my mother's angry voice, almost hysterical, when she found the stocks of foodstuffs which might have been kept and stored for future use, ransacked and sold off for next to nothing.

The men were being called up for war service, but luckily my father was drafted back into the steelworks, where he had spent several years of his life before I was born. Back at the lathe again, he was soon working thirteen, sometimes sixteen hours a day on essential war work. The school was temporarily closed, and one morning, possibly the very morning I should have been starting there, I went along with my mother to look through the railings at groups of miserable, crying children standing in the playground. They were about to be evacuated, and looked as if they had been rounded up, for each of them had a tag with their name and address pinned to them. It only shows what degree of panic and uncertainty had gripped people in those first months after the declaration of war, because a short time later we were to be inundated by an influx of kids from the East End of London.

Our family was entering a period of uncertainty and upheaval. The new house that we had moved into began to develop problems. You could say, it sprang problems – it leaked – it filled with water. The field at the back where we children played was full of springs. Maybe this is what had so attracted the snake, because there were frogs, toads and amphibians of all kinds in there. Every so often the cellar of our house would fill with water. And I do mean *fill*. I would sit at the top of the stone cellar steps and make paper boats, sailing them off on the dark waters that covered the coal and other things which we stored down there.

Again, this was fun as far as I was concerned, but a nightmare for my mother. I had no fear of the water, and felt confident that, if I was to slip off the top step into the dark water, I would swim or float with ease. She, on the other hand, was convinced that I would drown. I don't know who was right, but I can hardly remember a time when I wasn't able to swim. I loved being in water and felt completely at home in it. I was born a Piscean, after all! I don't know which weighed the most heavily with her, my imminent drowning or the fact that her prized piano in the parlour went mouldy. But one or both of these things drove us to leave home once again.

Luckily it was a rented house, so we didn't have the bother of finding a buyer. However, we didn't have anywhere to go and ended up living first with one grandmother and then the other. By this time a system of 'home schools', informal classes in neighbours' houses, was in operation, and my very belated schooling commenced.

* * *

War had been declared and people had been tensed-up and ready, but now there was a lull. After the initial fears and disruption which followed the outbreak of hostilities, people began to talk of the 'phoney war' and say 'it will all be over by Christmas'. Air raid sirens would sound from time to time, with their banshee-like wail, and we would leave our beds and scramble into the dark garden, groping for the safety of our new Anderson shelters. But usually, we would sit for an hour or so in this hole in the ground, trying to keep warm with candles and good humour, listening for bomb-laden planes which never came.

Youngsters were also on tenterhooks, either out of apprehension or anticipation of beginning their real school life, but then the tension relaxed into a situation which was neither one thing nor the other. Yet this interlude was deceptive: merely a prelude to the real war which erupted in earnest, causing much devastation to our city and our lives, in the next year.

Changes, though, were underway. Before long the real school opened up again (now that they had constructed underground shelters for us to bolt into in case of air raids) and I was soon trooping off with my small friends, gas-masks over shoulders, on that important adventure – school life. Father's job became more and more demanding as production was stepped up for the war effort, and we were still living cramped together in Little Grandma's small house. Then I overheard my parents talking about buying a house of their own. It was obviously going to be something special and different from anywhere we had lived before, because they sounded so excited about it.

It was now June, and I was six and a half years old on that unforgettable, sun-blessed day when we moved into our new house. While everyone was busy with the furniture and the unpacking and putting everything straight, I wandered off into the large, wild and unkempt garden. We were at the end of a cul-de-sac and the front gardens were very small, but they widened out in a fan shape behind the house, so that the back garden was huge. Running all along the bottom of the garden was a very old, dry-stone wall which had been the boundary to a country estate.

Although the house was relatively new, a thirties redbrick semi, the garden had been neglected by the elderly couple who lived there before us. On this midsummer day it was neck high in places with flowering grasses, and as I breasted through them they released clouds of pollen. As I pushed my way through brambles, I discovered blue carpets of forget-me-nots and violet and gold heartsease. I was thrilled to discover a few wild strawberries hiding in grassy hollows and an abundance of butterflies and other insects basking in the sunshine. Then there was an orchard of fruit trees with ten or more apple trees, six pears, four plums, and a plot of blackcurrant and gooseberry bushes.

After a joyful hour or so of solitary exploration, I was ready to go indoors and take stock of my own little bedroom and arrange my possessions. As the summer days continued, this wonderful garden became the focus for a lot of our activity. I don't know where the people in those wartime years managed to find so much energy and stamina, since air raid sirens had stepped up their frequency and woke us night after night. The men (and there were many men in our area who were working extremely long shifts in the steelworks) would spend the light summer nights and weekends 'digging for victory'. The women and children contributed equally their labour and enthusiasm. At first it was a heartbreaking wrench for me when my lovely wilderness of long grasses, forget-me-not-blue, and violet secret places, began to disappear under the determined spadework of my father. In some sensitive place inside I felt hurt by the destruction of this magical kingdom, but the growing-up self recognised the necessities and practicalities of life, and besides, I admired my father's work and forgave him. In fact, as the summer wore on, our relationship and bonding grew stronger and stronger.

With great patience he explained to me why we needed to make the earth productive, and what enjoyment we would all have when the ground was cleared and ready for fertilising with manure, and finally I could join in with the planting. By the autumn we were already harvesting our fruit and mother was busy bottling and preserving. Everyone, the whole nation, became involved in this exercise in survival and self-reliance, and I am convinced we became healthier and stronger for the exercise and good fresh food we had grown.

Our whole neighbourhood, and this also seemed to be reflected country wide, became caught up in a spirit of friendly co-operation. Garden produce was exchanged, so that those with a surplus of plums would swap a few pounds with a neighbour rich in runner beans or peas. The food available on ration in the shops was basic. Foul-tasting margarine replaced butter, eggs were rarely seen, sugar and sweet stuff, fresh meat and all the other things we had taken for granted, became extremely scarce. Manufactured foods like soup, jam or cakes were made out of indescribable rubbish, but we managed to get it down and survive.

Threats to our physical survival from another direction became an urgent consideration. We still hadn't been issued with an air raid shelter, and until we managed to get one, we would have to take some other measures. So another job for father was to construct a bomb-proof area in the basement of the house. We were fortunate indeed to have this spacious underground room, and at the back, between a strong wall constructed to support the chimneys above and another dividing wall, there was an alcove just big enough to build in two bunks. Father used some heavy timbers to support a big steel plate which he managed to fix above the bunks and between the two walls, and there we felt secure enough if a bomb should drop.

STORM

Thank God we managed to get this reinforcement done, and not a moment too soon. Air raid warnings were becoming a nightly feature. We lived and slept with the deadly droning of waves of bombers. Faintly audible at first, but inexorably drawing nearer until the sounds, vibrating in the sky, and echoing in the ground beneath, became something the ear attuned to, even in sleep. We would listen for the ack-ack guns to start up on the nearby hill, and feel faintly comforted, knowing they were 'ours'. We would listen for the reverberating wave to pass by each night, and learned from rumours that the German pilots had been ordered to drop their loads, not on us, but on the poor inhabitants of Liverpool and Manchester.

'Sheffield's been painted out with invisible paint,' 'Sheffield's on wheels,' people joked. 'Whenever they come looking for us, we just move somewhere else.' But silently, no one was joking. At that time the English Steel Corporation, where my father worked, had the only drop hammer in the country capable of forging crankshafts for our fighter planes. If that had been knocked out by a German bomb, where would our nation's defences have been then? Armour plating for battleships, vital parts for tanks, planes and artillery, not only for the British, but also for our allies, were in ceaseless production night and day by Sheffield's steelworkers.

Every sound in the sky summoned fearful alarms in the depths of exhausted sleep. Would this be the night? Or could we ignore the sirens this once and slumber on? It was now December and coming up to Christmas; it seemed very bleak and cold and people were worn out with work and unspoken fears.

* * *

Dad had given me a goodnight kiss and left the bedroom door open so that I could see the light from the landing, as usual. 'Hope we all get a good night's sleep,' he said. I woke a little later aware of a strange sensation. It was dark. Both my parents had gone to bed now, but I could hear them quietly talking. I called out to them in the darkness, gripped by a sudden uneasy knowing. Grumpily, my father climbed out of bed and came to see what was the matter. 'Dad,' I said, 'I was hearing strange sounds in the sky. It is like the planes, only I can hear them somewhere else. Inside me and a very long way off. They're coming for us tonight and something really awful is going to happen.' He groaned and told me to get back to sleep and not be so fanciful. 'What we all need is sleep, and not this nonsense.' He said it kindly but with fatigue and worn out patience.

Then it began. Far off and faint, but the sound was full of drawn-out menace. Black-winged evil: moaning, droning, thrumming its way through the cold, dark skies, and then the wailing rise and fall of sirens, as all over the city they began to join in. Shocking blasts of explosives shook us, as the bombs began to drop. We were out of bed, grabbing what we could in the way of warm clothes as we fled into the basement. Several unfortunate neighbours without shelters begged to come in too. Soon there were eighteen people crammed in together.

A ceaseless bombardment of incendiaries, parachute-mines and high explosive bombs fell from the skies, guns boomed and blazed, and Spitfires screamed overhead. Powerful searchlight beams streaked and criss-crossed the sky, and showers of exploding and burning metal could be seen falling to the ground. And for good measure, I was developing a high fever just to add to the inferno. I was burning up and had a raging thirst. Apparently, I became quite delirious and kept calling for water to drink. My poor father made several approaches to the basement door in an attempt to make his way to the kitchen to get water, but each time he opened the door a chink, a bomb dropped with an extra loud crash, close by.

The night passed. The sky was red from end to end with a hellish glow and ambulances were heard in the distant city, their sounds now joining with the noise of devastation. Then a silence descended and, in spite of themselves, people slept. In the chilly dawn there was but one thought in my parents' minds. We must get the hell out of here.

* * *

My father's brother Ewan lived with his family in a village close to Sheffield but over the county border in Derbyshire. By a miracle we managed to find a working telephone and warned him that we were on our way. Luckily our old car had a gallon of petrol in its tank saved for emergencies. This *was* an emergency, but it was also illegal to use a car unless on official business. So a plan was hatched. Big Grandma, who was showing signs of senility by now, had to be included in the evacuation, as well as Little Gran, and mother was detailed to pose as Big Grandma's nurse and was told to say that we were taking her to hospital, if we were stopped and questioned. Little Gran and I crouched on the floor and were camouflaged with rugs, so as not to be seen. Thus we set off to cross the city from the north where we lived, to Derbyshire in the south. But our journey was to take us into another bad dream. Everything familiar had disappeared. Roads were no longer there, buildings that had stood side by side in recognisable order were gone, and a heap of smouldering rubble replaced them. It was an appalling scene. Burned out buses and tram cars littered the streets, flaming gas mains and gushing water mains barred the way forward. Huge craters where land mines, with their massive high explosive loads had fallen and blown everything to smithereens, meant that time and again we had to turn the car around and try another direction.

Everywhere firemen, police and air raid wardens were dealing as best they could with the aftermath. The road surfaces were hot and a pall of smoke and steam hung above us. As we got into the centre of the city, almost every one of the big stores was on fire or a heap of debris. Big iron girders, which had underpinned the masonry, were now exposed like ribs of a carcass and twisted into monstrous shapes. The red-hot metal squealed and hissed, and it seemed to me that the familiar buildings were in agony. The all-pervading smell of burning lingered on in the town for years afterwards, and lives with me still in dreams mingled with the sound of those twisting, burning buildings.

Many hundreds of people had died that night and were still lying there beneath the rubble as we drove by. But we didn't know this yet and only guessed it might be so. At last we were out of the devastated city and climbing up into the fresh, cold air of the Derbyshire moorland, which we found to be sprinkled with pure white snow. How wonderful it was to disembark at last at the isolated house and be warmly welcomed by my Aunt and Uncle.

We had been expected, and there was a room, a meal and a fire awaiting us, but before long other relatives and friends who had been bombed out, appeared with their belongings and children. Everything now becomes confused in my memory. I was put to sleep in the big bed and I don't know what time of day or night it was when I awoke and someone noticed that I was covered in a bright, red rash. It was measles – and oh! what a wonderful way of repaying hospitality, to arrive with the plague, in a house now swarming with young children – and only ten days short of Christmas!

PASTORALE

We all recovered from the measles eventually, and managed to make Christmas both a celebration and a thanksgiving. My father went back home so that he could be nearer his place of work, and mother and I were soon the only refugees still left. This sojourn in Derbyshire was to become one of the happiest periods of my life.

I was now living in a large, half-built house in the countryside, and I loved it. My Uncle, I discovered, was never happier than when he was building, or demolishing and rebuilding things, and he was creating this house as he went along. He was making a long gallery, which was to be lined with oak panels and fitted with oak beams. You could have dismissed the enterprise as a fake, but the beams were genuinely old and so were the woodworm holes. Jacobean mullioned windows were already in place, with window seats, and the room was large enough to need two fireplaces, one at each end, to keep it warm in the cold weather. The final touch was a suit of armour placed to stand where its invisible, ghostly occupant could have a fine view out of the window and across to the distant hills.

The household was run on completely different lines from anything I had known before. A sort of organised, creative chaos. Buckets of sand and plaster, timbers and ladders, were strewn everywhere. The smells of these raw materials fascinated me, and looking back on this now, I am sure that my choice, many years later, to specialise in sculpture rather than painting, was formed through the smells and textures of plaster, wood and stone, dating from those days. I was probably influenced, too, by the rather more elusive atmosphere that the building activities generated: a kind of excitement at being involved in creating a structure that expressed one's individuality.

My Uncle had 'married up'. Aunty Belle was the daughter of one of the smaller industrialists, owner of a die maker's company in the city, and she had been a fee paying student at the Slade School of Fine Art in London. She was all 'fringes and beads' and arty ideas, *and* completely impractical. It was Uncle who bathed and changed the babies, and more often than not cooked the dinner. This was in addition to having a responsible managerial job in the same steelworks that my father worked in. He was also a gifted pianist, and had dreamed of making it his profession when he had been younger. The dreams had turned to hard reality, when he had to swallow the bitter pill of realising that a working-class family could not afford to finance the training for such a career. Maybe that was why this house, and subsequent ones, were somewhat over-endowed with pianos as a way of sweetening the pill. I think, at one time, there was one concert grand, one boudoir grand, one baby grand, and two upright pianos in various rooms. But he bought and sold them, rather like other men buy and sell motors. On one of these instruments, it was said, Chopin had played when he was staying at a friend's house, where the piano first resided. It was this very piano which my father bought from him and gave me for my eighth birthday.

I loved the house and I loved being surrounded by the countryside. There was some deep instinct in me which seemed to have an affinity with nature. I felt at home. Just as my mother longed to get back to her own home, I longed to stay where I was. Maybe it was here that it first began to surface, this difference in natures between my mother and myself. Something deep inside me responded to my Uncle's way of life. The house, the furniture, the pottery, the pictures. Perhaps, above all, I enjoyed village life. Walking down the lanes and across fields to get to the shops. I enjoyed sledging in the deep snow, and sliding over ice and frosty ground in the winter. And as winter turned to spring, my Uncle would take my cousin and me to look for the first traces of spring gold. Early catkins, and the bright yellow celandines and coltsfoot flowers which came before the leaves, and later as the sun grew warmer, there were primroses in the shelter of old stone walls. One day we went to visit a man who had a pet fox. He had it in a pen with a closed in section at one end. When he lifted the lid for me I could see, in the rather dark interior, this part-timid, part-fierce little face with big, inquisitive eyes. Wild and yet desirable it was, and it set me longing for a pet fox of my own.

TWO

FIRST MESSAGE FROM ASTRAZZURRA

I will now introduce my co-author. The Light, which I mentioned in the introduction as appearing to me in the darkest moment of my life, has become known to me as Astrazzurra, or Blue Star. This wonderful healing and guiding presence has become part of my life and instrumental in lovingly transforming it. Our partnership has developed and his communication has grown into a broader teaching and counselling role which, through the medium of this book, he wishes to extend to others. In esoteric circles, the term for such a spiritual teacher would be 'discarnate guide'. In my understanding, this term applies to an individual who has lived on Earth and has evolved through many lifetimes to a level where they are now dedicated to serving humankind. They make available the gathered wisdom of their own process and evolution through many lifetimes, and are also able to draw upon the combined wisdom of the group-soul of which they are a part. This is one of the teachings I received whilst writing these early chapters.

I am following your writing carefully and with interest. As you tell your story of your inward and outward journey, it will have meaning for many. The journey into yourself will have resonances for others which will strike chords, and it will be as if an orchestra of many instruments then begins to vibrate and harmonise together across the ether. This will have an effect upon the collective consciousness or unconsciousness, that place where we all 'touch' one another and become a collective 'body'. A body, not in the physical sense, but in the sense of the interaction and interpenetration of energies which make up the collective human psyche, which is the subtle body of humanity. We are all at one in the great sea – the collective unconscious. That great sea contains, not only our present consciousness but all that has been in our human story. All our deeds, and all our collective experiences are recorded in the great etheric ocean. It is the book of humanity.

We are etherically joined, we in the spiritual world and you on the material, physical plane. As these interconnections become stronger as our communication channels develop, a fine network is built up like a network of nerve pathways, and thus the whole body of humanity or its collective psyche is strengthened and can develop and go forward in its evolution. When momentous changes need to come about this great sea of consciousness needs to be stirred. We are at such a point of change right now. A new era is upon us and this requires a leap forward in humanity's conscious development.

We have come to that point now in our evolution where we are, as a mass, beginning to go forward into light. Moving away from the time-boundness and earth-body-boundness which has been the reality of our process until now. I am speaking even now in terms of linear time, because time is/was necessary to our learning experience on this earth plane. But as we go forward into light and lightness (which implies that the vibrational frequency of our particles will speed up) our bodies will also change. They will no longer need to be so dense in structure as we climb upwards to the mountain tops. As our vibrations heighten and the particles dance faster, we create for ourselves a lighter and lighter body material. This new body will be capable of extraordinary things in the future, of moving freely in space to other terrains without having need of the dense material and energy-expensive forms of transport such as you have at present, for instance.

Regard me as your friend and companion in the celestial quest for perfection, and as we travel further forward, these experiences of co-operation and communion between our two planes of existence will be more common for all people on Earth. Friendship and co-operation will be established between our two planes. The two worlds, which until now have seemed so far apart, will begin to come together in the not too distant future.

Until now it has been only through the death of the physical body that you have attained the heightened state of consciousness where you could begin to assess and understand the process of living in time and matter. It was necessary to shed the confines of the physical body in order to arrive at that place where you could have that perspective, as if from a mountain top, looking down and scanning the whole life which has gone before. Then free from the emotional entanglements, the power struggles, the every day concerns and obsessions which have prevented that calm and clear view, it was possible to see yourself and your mistakes in context and in a more objective, compassionate and detached way.

The story of human life has been one of great achievement and glory, but also of much pain, both inflicted and endured. Over and over we have become swamped in misery and fear, because we have not been able to maintain that clear view once we have descended to earth and become caught up once more in life's demands. For instance, a sense of *insecurity or greed has led to the amassing of wealth and territory. We have cheated and exploited and created that very imbalance in the divine order which would, if harmony reigned, manifest as the principle of abundance. We are here on Earth now, to restore that balance, to become healed, to become whole.*

Paradise existed on Earth. Your world, your Earth was created to be paradise, and this state EXISTS, present tense, because it always exists at the archetypal level. It is only at the level of time and at the material level that distortion comes about. Human existence is about the redemption of matter. We are the instruments whereby spirit comes into matter and matter is raised into spirit. This is what is meant by the coming of Christendom. Each of us carries deep within him/her self the Christ Consciousness and births it: we incarnate the Christ-Light each time we are born in flesh.

I am using Christian terminology here, yet of course you know that this light has been born by many 'Christophers' in Earth's history, Jesus and the Buddha are but two of the elevated beings who have carried the Light. The Light has incarnated on continents all over the world at different times to help illumine the way for humankind. Of course, the clarity and purity of the message has been distorted as it passed through the minds of earth-bound humans. The human brain as yet is an imperfect instrument of reception and perception. Yet each time a person takes the responsibility to meditate, to still the mind and allow stillness, peace and openness to flow into the heart, to let go the emotional turmoil and mental chatter for a while, then that stillness allows the brain cells to absorb more light. And then the instrument (the brain) changes, it clarifies, receives and reflects more of the perfected consciousness. Each of us then becomes a 'lighthouse' beaming out more and more light to fill the world. Our whole bodies then become transmitters and transformers of a powerful spiritual energy.

I will leave you here, for the moment, and allow your story to continue. But I would be pleased to be invited to join you and offer a further comment at any time.

BALANCING ACTS

Most cultures and conventions have tended to put human beings into strict categories – caste systems or class systems – and above all there is a strict gender category – we are either male or female. Any deviation from the culturally defined picture of what constitutes the role, characteristics or behaviour of man or woman, has usually met ridicule, intolerance and even cruelty. In my lifetime I have seen these strict distinctions soften at the edges and begin to dissolve, and witnessed a greater willingness to allow individuals the freedom to be themselves rather than copies of approved models.

In some ways, although I was born into what some would have termed a working class family, it wasn't until I was much older and had left Sheffield for London that I was made aware of the class system in this country. Our family, with its roots in a half rural, half industrial culture, included in it Great Aunt Laura, headmistress, trained singer and amateur painter, and Uncle Clem, who I seldom saw without a blackened face and back bent beneath a heavy tar-soaked sack delivering coal with his horse and cart. Then there was open-hearted Aunt Daisy with her overflowing proportions, greasy hair and dirty blue-white feet thrust into worn-out slippers. She lived in a run-down cottage swarming with innumerable children, yet she would offer me stale cake and hug me to her bosom like one of her own whenever I ran in to see her. I never knew my grandfather, he died before I was born, and although he was a steelworker the whole of his life, he also kept wicket for Yorkshire and for Sussex in the 1920s. Accountants and solicitors, lorry drivers and dustmen – all of this was 'family', and however disreputable or outlandish one member felt another to be, we all shared an unquestioning kinship – members of the clan.

We speak of the 'accident' of birth, but I would like to challenge that notion and offer another. The choice of birth. Consider the possibility that we choose our place of birth and we choose our parents. We are brought up in a culture which tells us 'You're only here once' usually followed by, 'so you'd better make the most of it.' This is often followed again by: 'Get what you can while you can, you're a long time dead.'

Our Christian religion has held out the promise of 'pie in the sky', good lives being rewarded by heaven, and bad ones by hell. But that is it! Death is a cut off point, the game is over and our score is totted up, and even if, in these recent times, most people have lost their belief in traditional religion or have become indifferent to its teachings, still the majority of us feel that *this* is the only life we have.

What a tremendous adventure opens up before us, then, if we realise that many of the incidents, accidents, encounters – joyful or disastrous – that we meet in this life, have been set in motion at other times and in other places by aspects of our Totality, our Being. Consider that we are a series of little selves, seeds from the Oversoul or Higher Self which drop to Earth incarnating fresh experiences in new bodies, different cultures, disparate eras. Then, history and geography are no longer dry academic studies. They become dynamic: the living, multi-dimensional book of our soul's education process. For the most part, for young souls, the process is unconscious, but as awareness strengthens over many lifetimes, conscious choice, and with it responsibility, comes more into play. The complexities and computations of all this are immense of course, and it is best, I think, to try to feel our way into it one issue at a time. The question of the choice of parents, for instance.

It may be very difficult sometimes to see why a particular choice was made. Often it would seem that we have made a bad mistake. But the choice was not made at the level of our present perceptions, it was made in accordance with our soul's purpose, and so that we could learn some important lessons, if we chose to do so. Could it have been my difficult relationship with my mother and the more positive one I had with my father, so that *he* was in some ways my true nurturer, that served to make me aware of the restrictions of gender stereotyping? A lesson perhaps in the appreciation of human uniqueness and individuality, free from the conventionally determined role.

I was well cared for as an infant and in my first two or three years I was closely bonded with my mother. She was beautiful in my sight, with her shock of thick, black hair and hazel eyes, all set off by our favourite emerald silk dress. I've never seen such eyes as she had. Gold, green and chestnut brown, all mingled together with a violet rim around the black centre. I would gaze into their magical, changing beauty as I lay cradled in her lap, every bit as enthralled as a modern child is by a sparkling mobile above its cot. I loved her passionately in my baby way, but as I grew older I felt a change taking place in her attitude towards me.

Protectiveness became over-protectiveness, and that in its turn became an issue of control, and then a battle of wills. Obedience was demanded without explanation or reason. With my father few of these difficulties arose. He was willing to listen to me and take my point of view seriously. He would reason patiently with me, and I responded without the need to rebel. I continued to be physically cared for by my mother, but although I couldn't have put it into words, I hungered for something more, and in those early years it was the two men in my life, my father and his brother Ewan, who provided it by nurturing my spirit.

As I began to reach out towards the bigger world, exploring and discovering what my being delighted in, my mother saw this as a threat. I was unlike her in many respects. My hair was fine and fair and curly, and my eyes were blue, and at first I must have seemed like a perfect little doll for her to care for and play with. But as I grew older she began to see me as a possession to control and mould into her own likeness. Every sign of her child having a character and identity of its own, she took as a challenge to her authority and a slight on herself. She became increasingly jealous of the time I spent in my father's company, and developed the idea that I was taking his side against her. All I was aware of in the beginning was a sense that she didn't love me any more, not as she had done when I was a baby. Something was going wrong with our relationship.

My father was soft hearted, outgoing and friendly, but as I grew older I was aware of my mother becoming increasingly intolerant and critical of people in general, and she made very few friends. She had her way of doing things and this was not to be questioned: it was law. She had no time for my arty aunt and she hated the mess and disruption that surrounded their unconventional and colourful lifestyle. She saw the mess, but somehow failed to see the beauty and the greater freedom that went with it. Or, if she did, it meant less to her than her own obsessive sense of tidiness and propriety. At one point we were all in favour of turning our two small downstairs rooms into one large one, and we began to plan how it might be, but as soon as it looked like becoming a reality, mother put an end to it because of the dirt and upset the builders might cause. Our menu was limited and boringly repetitive. Anything other than meat and two veg (very well boiled ones at that) was too fancy and dangerous: foreign messes. Food, it seemed, was the enemy and needed to be done to death. I was discouraged from being let loose in her kitchen for fear of what I might get up to.

Nothing was ventured, nothing dared. No risk, no change, no questions, no challenge, no self-examination. 'I am right, and you must do as I say because I am your mother'. This was the commandment which ruled the house.

As I write this, I begin to feel uneasy. These minor incidents, irritating though they may be, do not adequately explain the strong emotions I am beginning to feel inside my skin, down in my guts. It might be a good moment to 'tune in' to A.Z., as I often do when I am disturbed or stuck and need a viewpoint outside my own which will help me to see what I need to focus on. I pick up a pen and pad as I sense our contact beginning to flow, and I write down his words as they begin to form in my head:

As we come to this period in your life, and as you attempt to set it down, there is a perceptible tightening up in your body. Your throat, and your Throat Chakra in particular, are tense. There is much here to grieve over; you hesitate to express the feelings you have inside, and so the words don't flow so well. You are unwilling to expose your mother – to tell the world, as you see it, about her shortcomings and the pain and grief it caused you. I want you to put down just what you feel. I do emphasise feel.

Somewhere back then, I must have felt, though it wasn't conscious enough to be put into words, that if only I'd had a mother who supported my aspirations, my need for adventure, and encouraged me to open my wings and fly out into the world, then there wouldn't have been that build up of stress and unhappiness at home that made it feel like a prison. There were constant rows. My father was as much a target for her anger as I was. At times it felt as if a slow poison had leaked out from all the destructive words which had been spoken and seeped into the fabric of the walls. The walls no longer stood around us providing safety, but exuded a stifling miasma which we were forced to breathe.

No wonder my father found interests outside the home. But this caused resentment and jealousy, and more rows. I enjoyed being out and about with him because he encouraged me and nurtured my spirit of adventure. He opened up the world to me. It was he who taught me to ride a bike, to swim and dive, to play tennis and cricket. But he also helped me with my maths homework, and helped me to overcome the blockages I had developed through bad teaching at my junior school, where I had been walloped by the teacher for getting a few sums wrong. You often hear people say, 'I was caned and it did me no harm,' and I don't think it *was* the caning that hurt, so much as the injustice and the vindictiveness of the teacher who did the deed. I had a lot of time off school, around the age of nine or ten, because I had developed a tubercular gland and had to go to a clinic two days a week. I was unable to keep up with the rest in the tests we were given every so often. Being hauled out and caned in front of the class for getting a few sums wrong was humiliating. It did little to endear me to maths, either.

Dad was a good singer and was in great demand as soloist in the popular oratorios like *The Messiah* and *The Creation*, which were sung in halls and chapels all over the North. His friends persuaded him to take an audition for the Sheffield Philharmonic Choral Society. I remember him being very nervous about the prospect. Standing alone on the vast platform of the City Hall in front of a small panel of adjudicators, how small his voice seemed in the empty auditorium! Yet, not only did he pass, but he was put straight into the semi-chorus, which was a small section of singers who would be called on to do minor solo roles or more complex parts than the main body of the choir. My mother's resentment burgeoned again, however, and she began taunting him about spending his weekly night out with the 'Philandering Society'.

We shared this love of music, which must have been fostered in me from an early age, listening to my father's voice as he practised his favourite songs. The powerful timbre of his strong baritone as he thundered out the lines from 'Invictus': 'My head is bloody but unbowed,' or 'I thank whatever the gods may be, for my unconquerable soul.' The mellow, heart-stopping sweetness of what can only be described as a seaman's homage of love to his drowned companion in the song 'Tom Bowling', left a deep imprint on me. I learned to play simple piano accompaniments to these songs, and when Dad was accepted into the Choir, I would gamely struggle at the keyboard while he practised such adventurous pieces as Walton's *Belshazzar's Feast*, and Britten's *War Requiem*, or the early music of Monteverdi and Palestrina. My pianistic skills weren't really up to it – this was advanced, more difficult music, but we got a lot of pleasure simply out of attempting to create new sounds together.

People often dropped in. Neighbours, friends and relatives, knocked at the door and came in for a chat: this was our Northern way of things. Unlike the etiquette of the South, which I discovered when I left for London some years later, no formal invitations or introductions were required here. The women usually talked domestic affairs or swapped local gossip. They were 'outraged' by some trivia, such as that Mrs so-and-so, all tarted up, who had wheedled an extra ounce of meat out of the butcher, or was buying black-market butter off the ration. And they would utter disapproving squeals and wails: 'Eee–ey, I never!' and 'Did you see the way she paints her face? Ayh, it's disgusting!' I liked company and sat around anticipating that I would find some entertainment with the older women, but I usually became bored.

Sitting in on the men's talk however, was different. There was a lot of humour in their stories, and the room rang, not with disapproving wails, but hearty laughter. Listening to them, I became fired with enthusiasm for political and philosophical topics, and felt in sympathy with their social concerns. One of my father's great heroes at the time was Gandhi, though perhaps the West Indian cricketer, Learie Constantine, ran him for second place in this respect. Politics bored and irritated my mother, and she resented my interest. She seemed to interpret it as a deliberate stance against herself. Perhaps she was right to feel threatened and jealous. Perhaps I was usurping her place in my father's affections, but she pushed me further in that direction by asserting that her laws should be obeyed, when these laws were restricting, diminishing and downright humiliating. Or, perhaps it was her outbursts of weeping and rages, which seemed so irrational to me.

One incident comes to mind, which now seems greatly amusing, but at the time I felt shocked and hurt about it. It brought home to me just how much irrational jealousy must have been lurking inside her, and afterwards I never felt I could be quite so easy in my father's company again. During the war and long before televisions were thought of in our world, our one high point of the week was a Saturday night out at the local Picture Palace. It was usual for families to go together, and there was the extra treat of queuing up for ice-cream or orange juice in the interval.

This evening we set out in the blackout with our torch to walk down to the cinema, about fifteen or twenty minutes away. We walked along, all three of us arm in arm, happily engrossed in lively conversation. We laughed and chatted as we strode along with the torch light bobbing in front of us. But Mother became more silent, as Dad and I grew more animated. As we neared the Picture Palace, I could see we would have to pass a queue of people waiting on the pavement for the tramcar to town, and there wasn't room for us to get by three abreast. Unselfconsciously, I let go of my mother's arm, and father and I quickened our pace to walk in front.

We passed the queue and slowed down anticipating that Mum would catch us up, when she suddenly set upon us from behind, raining blow after blow on our backs with her umbrella. 'What on earth is that for?' we both cried in unison.

'Didn't you hear that?' my mother cried. 'That couple in the queue? That woman talking about you? "Disgusting!" she called you. "It's *disgusting*. Just look at that! That young woman arm in arm with that man. *He's old enough to be her father*!"'

I suddenly felt a lurch as an ugly image entered my head. It was a moment which precipitated me out of the warm, cosy innocence of childhood, and into another place where adults saw things differently and more disturbingly. Who was this flighty girl their adult eyes had seen in the dim light? Suddenly I was aware what they were imagining, though I hadn't known it until that minute. It was too soon to know it. I was in no way ready to see myself that way: mature and stepping into shapely, seductive young woman shoes. I'd never really wanted to be a girl, never mind a grown-up woman.

Yes. Do go on.

There was nothing to help me, during this prepubescent phase, to identify with the feminine part of my being. Growing up and becoming a woman was, for me, a completely negative proposition. Life seemed to belong to the male of the species. To the female, all was restriction and limitation. How often I was told, 'You can't do that any more, now you're becoming a young lady,' or 'It's all right for boys, they can look after themselves, but girls can't'. Boys can – girls can't, seemed to be the dominating commandment of my life, and not only from home but all around: from school, from magazines, from the radio and films. This became the focus for my own adolescent rebellion in the latter part of the forties and early fifties.

My father was all for allowing me much of the freedom he would have given to a son, but gradually mother wore him down. Her whole life seemed to become dedicated to wearing down both her husband and her daughter, until in later years, after I left home, Dad would escape and spend his days in his little shop at the other end of the city, nattering to fellow shopkeepers, customers and friends. (He had begun a new business by then, selling and repairing televisions and washing machines and suchlike.) He lived a life as far away from that atmosphere as he could manage.

When in my twenties and thirties I would visit him in his shop, he would confess to me: 'I just want to keep out of your mother's way. I can't bear to be in the house with her.' He went daily to and from that shop, although it wasn't making a penny profit in the end, until he was eighty five. It was as bad and as sad as that. When he finally gave up and retired, he had become stone deaf and fixed himself in front of the TV in the living room until bed time. He had ceased to be able to hear her any more and glued his eyes on the picture show in the box.

In fairness, I should have come in after your account of your mother wielding her umbrella, and stood you in her shoes – taken you into her psychology, and pointed out reasons for her emotional outbursts. Fears which she had of men and fantasies of sex as a ravening beast, which neither you nor she were aware of at the time. But I want you to have the opportunity to give vent to your own feelings, and for me to have interjected another point of view here would have stopped your flow. It was important for the flow to continue without interruption, so that the poisons of negativity could come out into the open. But after the expression of resentment and pain which has clouded your body and clung to you since those times, it is now time for some healing to come in. Time for reflection. Time for the light of understanding. Your mother was as much a victim of the times as you were, and also in need of healing. As new insights help you heal the girl that you were, you allow her to become healed also.

It was interesting, as you set the scene, that you depicted it in terms of night and dimness, and a torch light bobbing in the darkness. That was significant. We try always to live in the daylight. There we can cope, there we can use humour to help us lift out of potentially damaging situations and get along with life. And we get more and more skilful at daylight living. But the things we have assigned to the dark don't just go away, they live on, and things which grow in the dark take on some strange shapes. But you brought in your symbolic little light, which revealed to you some glimpses of the background and the family patterns which had produced the 'attack'. You were growing up and approaching puberty, and your mother had some problems surrounding that area in her own life. The area of emergent sexuality.

Unconsciously she feared that her husband was looking at you in that sort of way. She had many fears and fantasies about the male libido. She felt that men were obsessively driven by uncontrollable sexual urges, and might want to 'interfere' with their daughters. She had heard lurid tales. You know now that many of these tales are true. Many fathers have been 'guilty' of these acts which have devastated their daughters lives. Far more of this evidence is now coming to light which, in those days was unspoken, hushed up and censored. It was pushed down into the darkness and suppressed. As you three walked out that evening you were taking a journey through the local collective unconsciousness, with the help of a tiny bobbing light for guidance.

Your mother was afraid of sex and of men. Somewhere in her unconscious she saw a ravening beast waiting to pounce, in the night, as there it was at its most dangerous. She wasn't able to formulate these thoughts. There was no one she could talk to who could help her sort these things out rationally. They were taboo. One didn't talk about such things. Those who did were 'fast', 'a bad lot', one of 'those sort of women'. Respectable women didn't have sexual urges, lust. Men had lust, but that was something to be feared because it overpowers, sweeps away, and that brings down society's condemnation and revenge.

Sex, lust and sin were the three heads of the fearful beast waiting to *pounce. She saw your development into puberty as the beginning of this emergence – the beast raising its head – and didn't know how to cope with it. All the time you were walking and talking together, the fear grew inside her that sex was on the rampage, and in its most unspeakable form. It was, as it happens, a mistaken fear, and therefore her actions seemed irrational. If she had been able to speak about her fears and bring them out into the open in a more accepting climate, they would have taken a less overpowering form. By being unvoiced, the thoughts, images and fears remained in the darkness inside her mind, and so were all mixed up in an incoherent jumble, and that's what gave them such force. It came out in that attack on you both.*

But, as you say, at that moment all those years ago I was quite unaware of any of those images in her mind, and the attack was wounding. Not physically, and one could even see the comic side of it. But it snatched away the confidence I had in my relationship with my father, and damaged my sense of self, as well as damaging the relationship with my mother even further.

Yes, it wounded the girl that you were, and your feelings and emotions have held onto that wound ever since. Just as you have held onto other such wounds. But by allowing all this to come out, you are overcoming the resistance and the fear that your body has hung onto for all these years. By letting go, you are allowing new energy to be born.

You grieve for your father and for yourself and for your mother. You see what was created. What people can do to each other. What misery they can inflict, and how the potential for a loving, creative life can be stifled. And 'why', you ask, 'do we choose this scenario when we choose our parents?'

I gave this question some thought before writing down my reply.

REFLECTION

I am trying to understand that question as it relates to me personally. I can see how that 'choice' might operate in general terms. For instance, if in a previous life someone had grown up to become a brutish and insensitive father, it may have been necessary to choose a situation in the next life where that person could experience being an abused child so as to understand the consequences. But each individual case, when you start to look more carefully, seems full of complexity. Implicit in this, of course, is a belief in reincarnation. Each time we are born, the life ahead of us will be related to and a result of what has gone before. So there can be, if there is enough awareness, a growing sense of real purpose in our existence. At death we have the chance to assess our life from the higher perspective of the next world, viewing our mistakes and lost opportunities with a new understanding.

I believe that we are born on Earth to learn the lessons of material existence, and then we leave behind our physical body at death and go once again into our spiritual bodies. We gradually learn that spirit and matter are not opposed and separate, but are meant to be united. We are here to learn mastery. Mastery of the physical and the spiritual worlds, and that implies being balanced. All the dualities: good and bad, positive and negative, light and dark, need to be balanced from the centre point, and that centre is Love.

In order to learn this balancing act we have had many lifetimes on Earth where we have experienced imbalance. Every possible nuance of that experience will have been gathered into the total consciousness of mankind in time. The eastern concept of Karma is the vehicle of that learning process, reaping what we sow. Every time we have misused power, exploited a weaker person in order to gain more power for ourselves, exploited nature, exploited a People, for example, our karmic scales will have tilted, and caused us to be reborn in a position where we could, in the next lifetime, have experience of *being* exploited, and thereby regain our balance.

Yet, because we also have the gift of free will, some of us, some more than others, will have acquired such a taste for power that we will have become addicted to it and avoided learning the balancing act. Our debts will have mounted, our scales will have tipped further, until an accumulation of negative energy has so cloaked our souls that our chances of freeing ourselves of that heaviness get more difficult, and further away.

One of the greatest imbalances that has occurred on earth is that between men and women. At the Source, the Masculine and Feminine principles are in balance and harmony. I believe that we have many lifetimes where we experience life as one sex or the other in order to get the feeling of Masculine or Feminine as principles, but because of our taste for power the male has, throughout our history, become dominant over the female, and this is one of the lessons that we are only just beginning to address and get right.

There is also the balance of Positive and Negative to look at. First of all, as principles, and as they exist at the Source, there is no sense of one being good or bad, or one being superior to the other. They simply exist as they do in an electrical current, or as ebb and flow in the tide. Or, as we breathe in, so we breathe out. Bring it down to earth and see what happens when we begin to play the power game.

One human being wants to dominate and have power over another. Let's take the case of a husband and a wife. 'O wives, be ye submissive unto your husbands.' sayeth the priest (who is a man) and the husband thinks that sounds OK. So, sanctioned by the priest, he beats her when she won't obey. Getting beaten hurts quite a lot and she is soon afraid of him. Now the element of fear has come in, and power feeds on fear. In fact, the more fear you can create, the more power you can have, and the more disempowerment you have created. Now, man has created something which didn't exist before: fear. It begins to cling like a dark sticky cloud, around the negative pole. Once the balance has gone, the Divine Principles of Positive and Negative become distorted.

Meanwhile, the woman, who never asked to be put in this inferior position, still hankers after a status of self-respect and her own legitimate power. But she is now cowed through fear and her desire for power goes underground. Thus, the negative mother is created, and the power of the negative mother is beyond all imagining. She wreaks her revenge. Sometimes on her male children, whom she attempts to emasculate and tie to her strings. But more often it is her daughters whom she disempowers through her jealousy and possessiveness, using the weapon of her tongue, cutting and jabbing away at their self-confidence and self-respect.

And yet, this drama is not necessarily a tragedy, but more a powerful transformative performance. For without the villains and villainesses, the monsters and the witches, mankind's heroes and heroines could not emerge. Through our confrontation with our own darkness we have developed bright and shining strengths. And at the personal level, this confrontation with the negative mother, which is something we all have within us to some degree, provides us with something to struggle against in order to establish our identity as a person in our own right.

Coming down to Earth each time is like coming back to the classroom where we have the opportunity to learn important lessons. It also gives us the chance to try out a new role in a new production, with a new cast. Returning home to the spiritual world after we leave the body, is more like a holiday and a recuperation. We will have been given some guidelines there for our next appearance on Earth. We will have carefully chosen our main fellow players, but will we remember the guidelines once the unwritten play gets underway? We always seem to forget that we can have access to that guidance. If we want to develop that channel, that phone-line to our friends on the higher planes, then it can be done. What's more, they will be only too happy to communicate with us once again.

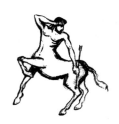

INTO THE TREES

I am sure that if I'd had reason to write about my life ten or twenty or even thirty years ago, a different set of memories would have come up at each point. All our records are stored inside us, in our psyche, and also in our body's cells. The wisdom within our psyche, if it is allowed to do its healing work, will release to our consciousness those memories and emotions which are relevant to the present moment. It is, perhaps, this growing understanding of the need to come towards a balance within myself that is stirring certain memories and bringing them up to the surface right now.

Eggy, with his fair, straight hair and clinic glasses is haunting me. We were the two idiots in the class who were caned that day for getting our sums wrong, and it was the pair of us again who were the victims of our teacher's wrath one afternoon when we returned, laden with bluebells from Whortley Wood. In the dinner-room one day he had suddenly said, 'Let's not go back to school this afternoon,' and I, struck by the brilliance of the idea no one had ever thought of before, said 'Yes, OK. But what shall we do instead?'

We decided to 'just go for a walk', and after disgusting dinners were over, we were let out into the playground. No one seemed to notice us picking our way diagonally through the mêlée of other kids towards the school gate and heading off in the direction of the park. In a few minutes we were through the park gates and setting out for freedom. We walked past flower beds, wandering further and further until we came to rough grass and the hill where skylarks rose up from tussocks and spired into the blue sky. Then our path grew steeper and we followed it down into a deep gully with a meandering stream below until it finally entered the shade of a quiet wood.

The scent of bluebells was all around us, there were white and pink campions, and school was far away in another world. We'd become enchanted; no need to speak. We each picked an armful of the richly scented flowers and uncurling, tender fronded ferns. We lost all sense of time. Wandering through the tangles in the green shade of the trees, our progress was slowed by brambles catching at our socks, or stilled altogether as we lingered in the warm patches of sunlight, listening to the woodland sounds. But after a while we found that we were gradually beginning to retrace our steps towards home and tea. It began to dawn on us, as we climbed through the lark tussocks and met the man-made world of brick paths and flower beds, that we would have to walk back past the school gates. What time was it? Surely school would be over by now?

In spite of the unease we were beginning to feel, the fragrance of the flowers still enveloped us in the magic of the woodland. Suddenly the furious figure of Miss T, our teacher, rushed at us out of the school gates. Eggy dropped his flowers and ran. I stood there transfixed and caught the full venom of the woman, who, with blazing eyes and flailing arms, lifted me off the ground and shook and shook me. My flowers scattered, my teeth rattled in my head.

This assault was inexplicable, but apparently we had played truant, which was very, very bad and we deserved what we got. 'Truant' was something new. It was all part of the mysterious grown-up world, and ours not to reason why. It was hard sometimes to make sense of why we were bad, but we had found out what happened to truants, so we didn't go bluebelling again. If the grown-up world, personified in this case by our Miss T, had felt able to explain rather than intimidate, then the young people in those days might not have felt so disempowered. Perhaps she herself had been ticked off by the headmistress who had put the fear of God into *her* by pointing out what might have happened to us in the wood, when we were supposed to be in her care. The Fear of God – this hierarchy of fear passing down the chain from on high – kept us in our place. Either that, or turned us into delinquents and rebels.

* * *

As I was in the midst of writing this, a rather strange thing happened. It helps to illustrate, I think, just how these new levels of communication and guidance, which I mentioned earlier, are beginning to operate. As our vibrations heighten we begin to notice a pattern behind everyday events, which we would have dismissed before. We find that we are becoming aware of how the world outside becomes a means of reflecting back to us just how much the universe is in tune with our thoughts and our needs. We notice a greater frequency of meaningful coincidences, or evidence of synchronicity (as the psychologist C. G. Jung called it) taking place in our lives. A leaflet, which my husband picked up unbeknown to me some days before, fell out of a pile of papers on a shelf. I pushed it back and it fell out again. I tried once more and it seemed to want to stick to my fingers, so I thought I had better look at it. It was advertising a workshop of the sort that is becoming more and more popular these days with people who are spiritually aware. It was devoted to the process of finding the path that will take us on our inner journey of self-discovery, back to our true centre where we can discover who we really are. It was headed 'Into the Trees & Finding Companions.'

In a little reverie just before this leaflet incident, the scene in the woodland, which I had just been writing about, had come back to me with such poignancy that tears had come to my eyes (an altogether rare event for me: I'm not a great weeper). I was surprised at the power of the memory and how strongly I had felt the presence of this friend who, until he spontaneously came up as a subject for the narrative, I had almost forgotten about. I was realising how innocent and true to our instinctive being we had been in those few hours we had spent together, and I caught myself saying out loud, 'Paul Eggerton, my dear, dead friend, I salute you as the *companion* of my childhood.'

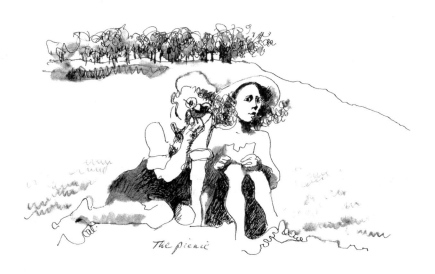

The picnic

DRAMATICS AND HISTRIONICS

While we were in the infant school, boys and girls played happily enough together, but once in Junior School we began to separate in our games in the playground. Being wartime, the big craze for the boys was zooming through the yard imitating fighter planes and having gun-fights, which was understandable enough, but they always seemed to end up in a heap of arms and legs on the floor punching and kicking one another. This didn't make sense to us girls, whose games were much more sociable and intelligent. Or so we thought.

Once away from the school yard, I would, more often than not, find myself walking home with Eggy who lived close by me. These journeys to and from school were never dull. We would soon fall into highly imaginative conversations inventing all kinds of fantasies. We could be practical too – we tied posies, made brightly coloured sugarless sweets, mystery packages, lucky bags, pea-shooters, all of which we sold to help the war effort. We organised nature-trail expeditions, bringing back tad-poles and strange chrysalises to hatch out in the school nature corner. We made costumes for the plays which we wrote, directed and acted in to raise money for hospitals. We were delighted to have an appreciative audience of grown-ups who actually bought tickets for our perform-ances. We became quite carried away by these amateur dramatics. Sometimes we managed to round up a group of younger children and allot them parts in the plays, but as often as not the two of us would dress up and play the parts ourselves. Princes and Princesses, wizards and fairy queens, haunted castles with horrendous apparitions on the battlements, dungeons with hideous skeletons of victims long forgotten, were our themes. But eventually our theatricals began to turn sour. Eggy became more difficult and temperamental, demanding that he should play the Princess and the Fairy Queen, and growing possessive about the dresses that we had made together. He became angry and emotional to the extent that we would come to blows over who would play the female lead. He would hit out and pull my hair, and I would hit back, where-upon he would cry and stamp.

I couldn't understand why he was no longer happy to play the wizard or some other suitable role. Why he felt compelled to compete for the dresses and the wings. Something wasn't quite right. Then, one day, my father came home from work and told me that Eggy's father had cornered him and spoken to him about his son. He had forbidden Eggy to play with me ever again because I was turning him into a lass. From hence forward, he was to play only with lads.

Of course we took no notice, but there had been a change. Eggy was often pale and quiet and frightened looking. The boys teased him and punched him – he didn't seem to know where he belonged. And I was losing interest. I liked roaming across the park with the girls, arms around each other in a crowd. Or I liked being out on my bike alone, shooting down the hills over the bumpy grass. It felt like flying. I dreamed often that I was flying, or galloping wild on horseback.

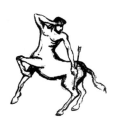

DIVISIONS AND SEPARATIONS

We were coming to the end of Junior School life and the eleven-plus was looming. This was the big exam which would separate the sheep from the goats,[*] in scholastic terms, for good. In those days, prior to the comprehensive system, we were divided by this exam into those who would go on to grammar school and become academic, and those who would fail and be relegated to the secondary schools where we would be trained for suitable employment in the sort of work which did not require much brain. All through school we had been streamed according to our position in class tests, and sat in strict order according to our results. There were five rows in our class and I seem to remember there were ten children in each row, which by my reckoning makes fifty children. We were the A class and there were the same number in the B class.

The A class were supposedly brighter than the B's, and the top row were the brightest of us all. I sat in the second row and our teacher had solemnly given her opinion that all the top row were expected to pass and most of the second row. One or two might just squeeze by of those in the third row, but that was very unlikely. So again by my reckoning, only twenty at the most out of one hundred children would become prize sheep. The rest, the mass, would be goats. The big day dawned. The day that we were to take this nerve-racking examination, and I went in clutching a piece of 'lucky stone' as a talisman, and a chrysanthemum leaf, because it had a wonderful, astringent smell which I could keep rubbing to keep me alert and give me confidence. Something about the arrangement of the desks, the new pens and pencils, clean inkwells and crisp new sheets of paper seemed to inspire me and I found that for once in my life I was enjoying doing the set work.

In the weeks before sitting the exam we had been given lists of grammar schools to make our choice from, should we be fortunate enough to

---

[*] '… and he shall separate them one from another, as a shepherd divideth his sheep from the goats. And he shall set the sheep on his right hand, but the goats on the left. Then shall the king say unto them on his right hand, Come ye blessed of my Father, inherit the kingdom prepared for you from the foundation of the world.' *Matthew 25, v.32-34.*

pass. The best schools in the city at that time, such as King Edward VII or the High School for Girls, were for fee paying students but they offered a few scholarship places to the brightest pupils in the exam race. But there were other very good schools to choose from and we were having a hard time making up our minds. My mother must have been touched by an angel, for she suddenly spotted one we hadn't noticed before. 'Good heavens, there's a Junior Art School,' she exclaimed, 'do you want to put your name down for that?' Of course I did, and I can only credit her with the vision which came to her at that moment. After making some enquiries, we found out that not only would I have to pass at grammar school level in order to get in, but that there was also a further special art examination to sit. Undaunted, I decided to go for it.

No one seemed to hold out much hope that I would be accepted. For one thing, the girls at our junior school hadn't been given art lessons for several years, although it was a subject I enjoyed and was quite good at. The boys had art classes, while we endured sewing classes instead, so I didn't fancy my chances too highly when I walked into the great hall of the City Grammar School where I was to take the art examination. I looked around the vast room, thinking I'd never seen so many children all in one place. A girl with tousled hair, sitting at the desk in front of me, turned round and winked at me. I smiled back. Papers and other materials began to be handed out. We were given a printed list of objects to select from and put into a composition which was to be drawn from memory. I sneaked a look at the other children around, and noticed a lot of worried faces, blank stares and shaky beginnings. Thin, dithery pencil lines and a lot of rubbings out. But my tousle-haired friend in front was going at it as if her life depended upon it. Thick, bold, black pencil marks were rapidly covering her paper, and as she worked and scribbled away she grunted. She was obviously enjoying herself. Her fingers and soon her face became streaked and smutted with graphite, and watching her with amusement, I lost all my inhibitions. I too went at it with zest and zeal.

Next we were given a real flower to paint, something I loved to do. Both Tousle-hair's painting and mine looked pretty good compared with those around us, I noticed, as the papers were handed in. Then came a group of objects for us to draw. Once again, the enjoyment of getting on with the work, and the stimulus of being given a still-life to draw, followed by a geometrical composition, neither of which I had attempted before, made me forget my nerves. By the end of the day I felt I had found my feet – my place – my heart. I knew this was what I was meant for. But then there were long weeks to wait after the exams were finished for the official envelope which would inform us one way or the other. At last it came, and the message it contained sent me to school that day floating on air.

The classroom was buzzing. Already, the ones wreathed in smiles because of their good luck were congregating together and talking excitedly. But, rather than showing resentment or disappointment, the 'failures' were also happily chatting together in groups and expressing relief that they would not be called upon, in their new secondary school over the way, to grind away at Maths and French, History or Latin, for the next seven years, under piles of homework. But I was to have the best of both worlds, for the Art School would require far less from us in the way of academic slog, because half the timetable would be taken up with 'glorious art'.

* * *

It was years later when I heard the news of Eggy's death. He had gone to sea after leaving school. Seeking intimate friendships with other men, he had become depressed by some rejection or humiliation, and jumped overboard.

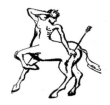

SECOND MESSAGE FROM A.Z.

As the story seems to have come to a natural watershed, leaving behind school companions and a phase of life, but not yet starting the new, I once again contacted A.Z. and invited him to make any comments he would like on what had been written so far. I never know what to expect, and this was unexpected.

I would like to comment, if I may, on what you were saying in your writing about your friend Eggy. Can I tell you a story?

He is present with me now, and I am learning from him of his interest and excitement at the possibilities which have opened out for him, and led to him becoming a healer. He has a strong potential for healing and a developing interest in magic. He is studying the healing powers of the plant kingdom and of nature in general; animals, birds, trees, rocks, crystals.

It is good to have contacted him again by your invoking of that woodland adventure. It is helping him, as it is helping you, to reconnect with that part of yourselves, and by so doing you will liberate those forces within you which have lain dormant.

He has had much anger locked up inside him, but he has been working on all of that and is able to express that anger in much more positive ways. As you know, we are working away on your blockages – your sacral and solar plexus* being especially blocked. This reflects the damage which was done in childhood years, since these two chakras are developing around the ages of five to twelve. Restrictions which were imposed by the adults around you were overwhelming at times, and prevented you from believing what your inner eyes could see, and therefore you were unable to be true to yourselves.

The prevailing climate at school and at home, blocked out for you the possibilities of extending your true perceptions, so that you were not

---

* A.Z. refers to the Solar Plexus and the Sacral chakras. These are two of the classical seven chakra system, comprising Root, Sacral, Solar Plexus, Heart, Throat, Brow and Crown chakras. See Appendix for a full description, and the diagram on page 234.

even aware of what was going on. You were very much drawn to the magic of nature and had real potential for learning its ways. Listening to the trees, being in the heart of the forest, you could have connected with the wisdom of nature that surrounded you – the spirit of the place was yours to command – and still is. It called to you but you blocked it out and shut the door on it. It was a thing so alien to the grown-up world, and they were dragging you in the opposite direction.

They were doing their duty, as far as they were concerned, in educating you in the ways of the world, yet such an alien world to your natural child spirit. It was all very necessary. You could not be allowed to become wild, uneducated, uncivilised creatures; heathen children of nature, as they saw it. So you were imbued with the Bible and its forbidding aspects. God was made into a fearful overseer, watching you from on high. Looking out for all your sins. Sexual curiosity was forbidden and a sense of sin was inculcated. Your poor friend Eggy was so disturbed that he took the only way out to him at the time, and drowned.

The sensations you are experiencing now in your body, as you write this, are sympathetic. You are sensitively feeling into his predicament, which was linked to yours. The misery and depression, which led him to take his life, cloaked the burning anger that he felt at the injustices he had suffered. The outbursts you encountered were part of that, but you couldn't know what was going on beneath the surface for him – at home mainly, but all around. The example of that macho father – so opposite in character from himself, despising and ridiculing the sensitivity and femininity of the boy, was too much to bear. He tried to escape – to the great sea – to wash it all away.

But now he has learned to understand his anger and to release his sense of guilt. His life goes on. You have parted and it seems, for you, a great gulf of time to cross. Yet he is near as we speak. He sends you love and good wishes and he wants to help you with your task of letting go the past which binds you and blocks you. You share some of the same work, since you shared some of the bad experiences which created the blocks. Through the act of imagination or visualisation, you can create a potent healing arena. If you will, arrange to meet again in that woodland, only this time it will be on the inner level.* He can bring in the healing foci: he can create the trees, plants, formations of rock and stone, flows of water and air, infiltration of sunshine, warmth of wood fires, in fact, all the elements that, combined, will enhance your healing journey.

---

* The outer world is physical reality. The inner world is our personal psychological territory which we can train ourselves to perceive. Working with this dynamic brings healing into our life.

And in this place messages will be sent – signs and signals will be discovered, pointing you in the right direction as you pass through the trees. He has friends in the animal kingdom and uses them as messengers to bring down his thoughts to Earth. There is a magical circle, already set up, of sacred stones. He asks you to enter and sit in the stillness, and all the healing elements will combine to bring you well-being.

Much love goes with you – Angelic and Earthly love.

Heartsease is yours again.

This last sentence, 'Heartsease is yours again', I first took to be a rather poetic way of saying that healing would come for my heart centre, and for the pain and grief that it was carrying. Also, it seemed to be a reference to the fact that I had spoken about my delight at finding masses of these wild flowers, with their blue and yellow, violet and gold hues, in our garden when we moved into the new house. But it struck me a little later that there might be yet another layer of meaning intended – with a rather unexpected touch of humour – when it dawned on me that heartsease was another name for wild pansy.

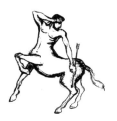

THREE

from The Tyger

On what wings dare he aspire?
What the hand dare seize
the fire?

William Blake 1757-1827

BUDDING ARTISTS

The next year brought jubilation for the ending of the war, and saw the citizens of Sheffield organising victory celebration street-parties. It took me to my new school in the centre of the city.

My new green blazer bore a badge that sported an array of initials: an embroidered JAD surmounting a shield with SCAC emblazoned below. It proclaimed the bearer of the decoration to be a member of the Junior Art Department of the Sheffield College of Arts and Crafts. A hand-me-down, but nevertheless top quality gymslip, courtesy of one of my Leicester cousins, completed the outfit and launched me into the grown-up world. Travelling every morning on the tram with important people on their way to work in the city, I was going somewhere too.

The proud Victorian edifice which had originally housed Sheffield's art students was now just one bombed-out shell among many others. We juniors were put into makeshift classrooms next door, in a building which had once been a factory of some sort. Across the street we could see the back of the Lyceum Theatre, and around the corner was the Egyptian inspired, Portland Stone edifice of the City Art Gallery. Below us, steeply sloping away to Pond Street, was a vista of blackened ruins – shattered walls of roofless houses with shreds of flowered paper clinging to them, firestruck workshops, pubs, shops, cinemas, in a mass of rubble and twisted metal.

On that first morning, as I struggled to take in all the confusing impressions, I spotted Tousle-hair sitting in one of the desks in our first-year classroom. We formed an immediate bond and became allies. Before long two other new girls joined us and we became inseparable companions for the next four years. However important that adolescent bonding proved to be, it was the strangeness and unfamiliarity of our surroundings which made its impression and overawed us at first. The view right outside the first-year classroom window, so close that it seemed to be looming in on us, was of massive contorted iron girders, tottering brick walls and the charred timbers of perilously caving-in roofs. Devastated buildings over which the smells of burning still hung.

All these bombed buildings were ruled strictly out of bounds, so we took this as a challenge and spent our lunch hours climbing in and out of these death-traps, hopefully unobserved. We smuggled illicit tobacco and cigarettes, lifted from our parents' pockets, and had smoking parties in the burned out wreckage. We crawled through underground tunnels and ruined basements. We made secret caves in the rubble and crouched amid ashes and charred timbers exploring the mysteries of sex, menstruation and childbirth. Alternatively, we terrified one another with ghost stories and supernatural enigmas. When we tired of this cramped and lurid atmosphere, we challenged each other to more and more difficult physical exploits. Climbing up to an upper floor of the ruined old Art College by means of the bits of iron bars protruding from the wall where the main staircase had once been. Or crawling through tiny spaces into a dark underground room to reach a six-foot long wicker trunk which we could dimly see half buried in dirt. Just big enough to hold a body! The fact that it did indeed hold the remains of the skeleton from the anatomy class well repaid our thirst for horror.

There was no playground in our make-do school, and so our teachers had no option but to let us wander the streets in the lunch-break. This was an education in itself, as we got to know the characters in various small shops and workplaces. There was the woman who sold slices of bread and jam for a ha'penny. Jam and *butter* was a penny. A few yards further down the street was a blacksmith's where we congregated in the arched doorway, dodging the sparks and coughing from the smoke and acrid stench of burning hoofs, while we watched great shire-horses and dray-horses being shod.

We discovered, among the narrow streets of half-bombed, half-standing buildings around the school, the dark and crowded workshops of the 'little mesters'. There, in the dim interiors, old men crouched over sparkling grinding wheels or flaming forges. They fashioned blades of complex penknives or beautiful cutlery sets with loving care. They didn't speak; they worked away in silence, knowing we were there all the time. After a long, patient while we would be rewarded with a gruff grunt and a warm, sooty smile.

One of our discoveries was a buried hoard of mother-of-pearl. Thousands of magical fragments of this treasure we dug out of the burnt ground with our fingers, unearthing iridescent, sea-lustred buttons, shimmering flowers and tiny carved figures. There were also rough, unfinished handles of mother-of-pearl and ivory which had been meant for those very knives which the little mesters were still producing. This pearl factory had employed women workers, and it seemed fitting that these handles were intended to be coupled to the steel blades crafted by the men.

A curious afterthought I must record at this point. I have had, at intervals ever since we unearthed that treasure, dreams of digging down through layer after layer of strange incinerated earth, then coming upon wet sand and finally, pools of sea water. And finding at each succeeding layer the most extraordinary, numinous, minutely sculpted figures. They were vaguely reminiscent of Palaeolithic figurines found in the depths of Cretan caves, yet alien. Different enough to seem to have come from another planet altogether. Tiny forms of great power, yet unrecognisable as anything I have seen on Earth in this lifetime. What this was telling me, I still haven't fully understood.

Our Junior Art School was a small and very unusual establishment. When I joined there were only three classes – first, second and third years – with twenty-four pupils in each class. The school leaving age was fourteen. When it was raised to fifteen, another room was found for us in the old factory, and one more teacher engaged. At first there had been four teachers; the headmaster who also took mathematics, geography and a smattering of science, a woman who took us for English, history and French, then two more women teachers who taught art. Because a much greater proportion of our time was taken up with art lessons our formal education was minimal, so we were not following the usual syllabus leading to the equivalent of O level or A level. This was not for us. It was expected that some of us would leave at fourteen or fifteen with the ability to draw well enough to find employment in one of the city's firms as a designer, and others would be selected to go on into the Senior Art College and perhaps become painters or sculptors.

In 1945, the thinking was that creative artists would make their way to prominence in their own field by their innate talents or genius, and those who fell by the wayside didn't matter anyway. But that view was reversed later when art students were accorded degree status at the end of their training, and so had to provide themselves with the right background of O and A levels before they were accepted onto the degree courses. Then these idiosyncratic junior Art, Music and Drama departments were left high and dry and had to close down.

I have often wondered since whether my lack of exam-oriented teaching was an advantage or a disadvantage. I have to admit feeling, by the world's standards, to be under-educated and at a disadvantage in many ways. There has always been ambivalence in the way our British culture has regarded artists and art education in general. It is not at ease with such people, I think. Artists do not fit neatly into conventional categories.

In the end I have to conclude that what I gained from this unorthodox little school far outweighs what I may have lost. It was far ahead of its time in the way its boys and girls were merged together. On the sports field for instance, there were such a small number of us that we could only muster one team of girls for hockey, and one team of boys for football, leaving over a gaggle of assorted genders to play, one week mixed football, the next mixed hockey. Needless to say these mixed games were hilariously unserious. As were the occasional bouts in the gym of a game of Rugby Touch. We girls discovered that as soon as one of the boys gained possession of the ball we could grab his shorts and hold tight. He couldn't run or even throw without the danger of a red face and lost composure. These tactics achieved some equal scores.

Art school life was rich and interesting. Not only was there tuition in drawing and painting, lettering and script, but there were the craft workshops where pottery, silversmithing, woodwork and dress designing were offered. There we met older students from the Senior Art College who seemed very mature and sophisticated. Interesting and fulfilling as our school days were, the over-riding experience for many of us came at the end of the second year when I was thirteen. We boarded the train for Grantham, I with my father's ancient bike, a 1920's Raleigh, stowed in the luggage van, and embarked on three weeks annual farming camp to Lincolnshire.

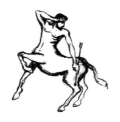

A.Z. THIRD COMMENTARY

I am beginning to realise that asking A.Z. to comment from time to time is going to be more of a challenge than I had bargained for. I am constantly surprised by the unexpected nature of the input from these higher levels of consciousness from which he speaks. It is not only the nature of the teachings, but it seems my own education, spiritually and psychologically, will form part of the exercise. I am always given the choice of how far I want to go in this matter, needless to say.

You have mentioned dreams, and as you know, they are an important line of communication. The language of dreams is one of the ways in which that which is hidden, or beyond and below everyday consciousness can express itself. Dreams can reveal to us parts of ourselves which we have lost or forgotten. And of course, we can also retrieve material which we have shut out and pushed away into our unconscious, at times in our lives when this stuff was too difficult or painful to cope with. But as long as we are carrying around repressed material there will be energy locked away within it, energy which isn't available to be used positively.

So! You know all this. But do you also know that the vital communication energy of dreams flows from the Astral planes and carries messages from there? Everyone receives input from those planes all the time, though they may not be aware of it. Dreams are most important. It is through this element or medium that we communicate our longings and desires for you. I do not mean sensual or emotional desires, but our desire for what we would teach you of the world which is to come – the future world which you may inhabit – and you also communicate with us your longings and desires.

Dear friends, we come to you on wings of longing and delight. Delight at what you have accomplished so far on the Earth plane. We are longing to meet you and talk with you and give you great joy, and tell you great news of all that is in store for you.

You are wondering what is coming next! I am here to tell you much. I am listening to your voice Esmé, as you tell your story, and it is in deep thought that I reply.

Looking back at what we said previously about the boy you called Eggy, and how he has learned to release that fiery anger – and linking that to the fire scorched earth that you have recently described, I want to teach you something in this. It rests upon an act of war and a betrayal of security. We each need security in our lives in order to grow strong and true, and those who destroy that security, in whatever manner – in the home – or in the wider context of the destruction wrought by war ...

I broke off at this point with some astonishment when I 'heard' a voice, seemingly from inside myself, complete the sentence by saying, 'are wicked and they must be punished utterly and with great severity.' I was so taken aback that I was in doubt whether to go on. This wasn't the voice I was familiar with! These weren't the sentiments of the patient, unconditionally loving guide I knew! I steadied myself, quieted my mind and emotions, and focused my consciousness back again at the level of higher mind (Brow Chakra) which I need to do when I contact A.Z.

You have just heard a voice from your own psyche talking of punishment. How will you learn to distinguish the voice of your true teaching source from other voices coming from your unconscious, what we might call sub-personalities? You see there are pitfalls in the receiving of guidance and one needs to be wary and able to discriminate. Let me try to help here.

We were speaking of fiery energy and anger and of war, when you heard a voice from within you speaking of punishment for evil doers. You had changed the focus of your attention, as you switched from listening to me, to writing down what you had heard, and the level of your focus dropped and with it your vibrational energy. It is easily done. The fiery energy was building up in you and was releasing from inside you, and within it were some demons and monsters who were willing to come out and confuse you – hoping you would take their voices for mine. Don't be afraid. Let them come, let them speak. They speak of punishment for evil men, of wrath to be metered out. Breathe calmly and focus into your Brow Chakra and the level of vibration there, it is blue and clear and holy.

There are demon voices within you and they are aligned with the God of vengeance and hell-fire. This is the negative face of mankind's image of God. There is in man's consciousness, in the collective unconscious, a God of hell-fire and destruction, which has been implanted down the ages. It goes very deep. It is a most powerful archetype. Feel that energy within you, feel its force. You are carrying a lot of that consciousness – mankind's wrathful God of vengeance. What will transmute it?

First of all, be aware of it. You have contacted fire and let it loose.

Now let us turn to the healing aspect of that same element, and to the conversation we had about Eggy and his healing circle. He also has had a great fire stoked up inside him – burning him away. The fires of hell consuming him. His own anger turned to vengeance towards those who betrayed him, both in this life and reaching back into other lives.

Take heart. This is a progression in our contact. If you will allow yourself to be used as a guinea-pig in this way, in order to show (your readers) how negative material can be transmuted and transformed. It is your choice, to say yes or no.

The fire energy comes up from your intestines and is consuming you. You have been hurt and the god inside you seeks vengeance. Feel the calm, blue energy from the Brow Chakra, that level where we meet one another. Feel it flowing downwards and meeting that fire in the guts, and in the solar plexus. Feel it pouring its sweetness and calm into the core of molten hate inside you.

At this point I became aware of my Brow Chakra opening to its fullest extent and what felt like a cool blue waterfall of light and energy pouring out of its centre and flooding into my body. All inside my abdomen and the area of my solar plexus. That part of my body felt hot and tense and knotted up. When the blue light flowed in, it did indeed feel as though clear, cool water was being poured into a crucible of molten lava with the strangest sensations resulting. I focused on my Brow Chakra again and waited for the message to continue.

And now you see, the explosions begin! A wonderful display of fire-works, a rainbow of colourful stars! The sparks fly. The grinding wheels come into play and old men chuckle as they work, fashioning beautiful tools. Knives of wit, keen edges for defining clarity and cutting away dead branches. Surgeons' knives for operating with skill. We shall have a display to marvel at. All is incinerating but it leaves behind a clean wound ready to heal. Let the burning take place, but enjoy it. Let the tools be sharpened, burnished and polished. The old men are setting to, and greeting their new task with alacrity. There is much merriment.

Let the wounds be red and healthy and no longer festering. Let grace begin. Let carnival commence. Celebrations are in order, when the wounds are cleansed of their poison.

I am with you now in joy and peace. We can dance and be merry together my love. My ever-one-with-all in love and light together.

That was a remarkable interlude – and quite unexpected, was it not? There is much more I would like to tell you about the destiny of places and peoples, and why certain people were drawn to a place such as Sheffield, as an example. But perhaps you need to digest the experience you have just had and you might invite me to return again a little later.

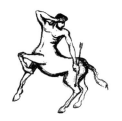

SWEET THIRTEEN

We were met at Grantham station by War Ministry lorries and by strange German accents. Fair haired men in heavy boots and cotton khaki uniforms with POW stamped everywhere upon them. Although the war was over now, prisoners of war still remained here in great numbers and were being put to work helping with the harvest. It was my first encounter with one of the 'enemy', and thrills ran through me. For many of us, this train journey was probably the first in our lives which we had made without parents, and the high pitch of excitement at landing in this strange place amid all the sounds: doors slamming, whistles shrilling and steam snorting from the engine, was mixed with alarm. Were we all complete? Where was our baggage and has someone unloaded our bikes from the guards van? And now there were these strange foreign accents and a fleet of lorries drawn up waiting to take us away. The fact that they were powerful military looking vehicles with 'Kestheven War Agricultural Executive' written on them, confused me, and for many years I thought Kestheven was a town in Germany.

I don't know where I thought we were being driven off to, but we were soon racing through the Lincolnshire countryside in warm afternoon sunshine. Passing by open fields, groups of young people like us, or gangs of supervised POWs, would stand up, pausing from their work in the fields to wave to us, and our driver would yell and hoot his horn and wave back. Then we began to slow down as we drove through tree-lined lanes, and finally turned into a private driveway and came to rest before a beautiful old country house.

I was thirteen and something of a tomboy still, and here we were in a requisitioned country mansion: boys, girls, young men and women (for some of the older students from our art college were there too) all living together in the countryside in midsummer. There were haystacks to romp and roll in, and a romantic walled garden with espalier apples and peaches. It was hot, and everywhere there was this heavy, sweet scent of honeysuckle and ripening corn; and mingling with the sensuous fragrances were the all pervasive sounds of that most optimistic, energetic musical Oklahoma. Spilling out from radios and gramophones everywhere around us came its affirmative message that the 'corn was as high as an elephant's eye,' 'a bright golden haze was upon the meadow,' and 'people will say we're in love'.

Then of course there was the work. Hard, heavy, backaching work in the fields. We were driven to and from the outlying farms each day by Sigmund, one of the German prisoners, and our headmaster, being the sort of person he was, encouraged us to get to know this young man by getting permission for him to join us each evening after work. Sigmund ate with us and became a hero to the young boys by regaling us with stories of his youth in the Black Forest, where his father was Captain of Forestry. It turned out that he wasn't German after all, but Czech. We would all sit out on the veranda discussing the war and the present political situation concerning the imminent carve-up of Europe into communist dominated areas and the territories allotted to the Western allies. Sigmund was afraid of returning to his homeland, since it seemed inevitable that his town would fall into the communist ruled territories when the maps were drawn. As much as he disliked the Germans, for he had been drafted into their youth army around the age of sixteen when his country had been overrun, he feared the Soviets even more.

Coming back from the fields each evening in the speeding lorry was a thrill. It was a high sided, canvas topped affair, and we rode standing up, holding on to the hoops of steel which supported the canvas, while the wind whistled through our hair. The lorry would sweep off the road and into the half-mile drive up to the house. Sigmund would turn a half-circle in the yard before slamming on the breaks, and we would wait for him to get out of his cab and stride to the back of the lorry to help us down. The boys happily grasped his strong arms as they leapt over the side, but some of the older girls would feign feminine frailty, pretending their ankles might break if they jumped from such a height, and they would slither over the side showing thighs and knickers. I scorned this display, but one day, as I sprang from the back of the lorry, his arms held me suspended. With what seemed to me astonishing strength, he held me in the air. We turned around and around in a slow pirouette, then he brought me gently and tenderly down to the earth and closer and closer towards his body, so that when my feet touched the ground there was not a hair's breadth between us. I closed my eyes, my heart melted and I was gone.

The dormitory I shared with seven other girls was quiet and peaceful as I emerged in the early light of dawn the following morning from the sweetest dream. Naively and sleepily I whispered to my friend in the bunk above me, 'I was in the woods with Sigmund and we were picking bluebells. There was the most wonderful, delicious feeling like I've never felt before.' There were sudden hoots and shrieks from the rest of the dormitory. 'You soppy idiot,' they shrieked, 'you're in love. You're in love.'

I went down to breakfast, collected my thick piece of bread and fried egg, and sat down at one of the long wooden tables. I chose a seat alone in a patch of sunlight feeling the need to be solitary, as the dream sensations still clung to me. I felt slightly woozy in the way that you do after a glass of cider, but it was different – magical – and I didn't want to join in the noise and chatter of the others. I felt anxious, although I didn't know why. I kept watching the open doorway from the kitchen. Then Sigmund came in, and I knew why I had been on tenterhooks. He looked round the room then slowly walked over towards me and sat down.

Everyone noticed his entrance and soon several others came over and joined us. I was no longer alone and the magical spell gradually dissolved. Yet his presence beside me gave out warmth and strength. He smelled of clean cotton and rare unguents. The Nivea cream, which he rubbed into the skin of his muscular arms, was not only a luxury substance in those times, but no self-respecting British male would have deigned to use it. Yet this exciting alien creature spent his precious allowance on preserving his body and enhancing his tan. His white teeth gleamed as he smiled at me and the fragrance of honeysuckle drifting in from the window was overpowering.

He had this immense courtesy and politeness. He gave his full attention to everyone without favour, yet he kept turning to me. He asked if I was staying on to the end of the three weeks of the camp. But I told him that I was going with my family on holiday, so I would only be there a couple more days. 'I also will be returning soon to Germany,' he said. 'Please would you like to write to me. I shall be lonely when I get there. This has been the most wonderful experience for me to have met you all. I have never before known a more wonderful headmaster and group of school children. It was not like this for me at home. How fortunate you all are to have this caring and freedom. It must be always for you, lessons with a joke and a smile.' So we exchanged addresses, and I held his piece of paper tight and wished that he would kiss me there and then.

In a few days my parents came to pick me up me in our little car. We had planned to go on holiday to the south coast after farming camp finished. I excitedly ran to greet them and grasped my father's hand, dragging him off to meet Sigmund, the most wonderful man in the world. They came face to face and Sigmund stood up straight, saluted and clicked his heels, declaring, 'I am very pleased to meet you, sir, the father of this lovely daughter.' I'm sure he thought he was making a gracious speech, but Father's demeanour changed, becoming a spluttering, inarticulate iceberg. Later in the car he said, 'What was I supposed to say to him. We've just spent five years fighting these buggers, these blighters. And you're only thirteen!'

* * *

Sigmund did indeed write to me after the new school year started, and I have his letters still, in a box with those of other friends and sweethearts. The letters faded over the years, but the poignancy of that first love faded even sooner, as the demands of life began to quicken pace. There were tests and exams at school and there were crushes and infatuations. But though these romantic encounters with callow youths were more appropriate to my age, and slightly more acceptable to my father, yet nothing stirred my soul nor came close to the poignancy of that first affair of the heart.

Another two years and our time in the JAD was coming to an end. Some of us were drawn by the prospect of becoming independent and earning our own money, and jobs at that time were plentiful. Others felt the call of an artist's life and went hopefully to interviews for the Art College proper. We seemed to have selected ourselves, as the putative bohemians all got through their interviews and were accepted.

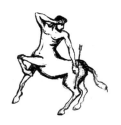

A.Z. FOURTH COMMENTARY

I sense that we are about to come to another threshold in your life. This time, a visionary opening out to new scenes and vistas, but I think we need to pause here awhile before you rush through that door. Can we come back a step – to the farming camp episode.

It was a wonderful period of great development. Physical strength was gained and health was invested in, and your heart was free from pain. It was a moment to treasure. Spend some time now to go into it again – relive its peace and promise. That moment when your heart felt love. It was such a brief encounter, it lasted for a moment and was gone. Draw it back and relive it: let it expand.

You haven't been able to open to that moment since, because of the sense of shame you felt when you exposed your heart's feelings to others. Even though it was meant as fun, the girls shattered that sweetness with their ridicule: a laughter which belied their own emotions, perhaps of jealousy, perhaps embarrassment at their inability to cope with delicate and tender feelings. And then there were the even more powerful emotions of your father. Completely understandable emotions of protection for his young daughter whom he thought was in danger of being taken advantage of by an older man. Not only that, but this man was one of the hated enemy. All this caused a closing up of the heart which had felt the quality of love.

There are tender and vulnerable moments which need to be allowed to blossom. A bud needs to open gently, but it was not given that chance. A fragile and delicate flower was about to open and was subjected to a chill storm, which caused it to shrivel. You think maybe I am making too much of this, but I am trying to demonstrate something important. The awakening of Love is, perhaps, the most important lesson for humanity at present, as it is this energy which will raise up our vibrations to that level necessary for our transformation. Humanity's Heart Chakra needs to be enlarged and opened so you can receive and pour out love to one another as you journey into light.

If the tender heart is assaulted, what chance has it to grow and bloom? Many hearts are shrivelled in the storm or the burning sun before they can become firm and beautiful and capable of bearing perfume to the world. But you now have the opportunity to heal your budding heart, and everyone can become healers of their own damaged hearts, because each one of you can take that journey backwards into your own lives, becoming the parent to the child within you. Loving it and nurturing it as it was never loved before.

Heal the moment, heal the past. Love was awakened within you at that tender age, in your case by this handsome hero, and we will all have a prince or princess charming of some kind who kissed us awake. Yet the mistake we all make is to assume that the gift of love lies with the person who awakens that passion. We open a window to the truth and the light when we open our hearts. We let love filter in and it drenches us while we sleep and fills us with its fragrance. We should bless the person who opens that window in us, but keeping it open is our responsibility.

I would like to open up and share with you the mysteries of Love, but it can't all come at once. Awakening to love, one is aware of an enhanced beauty and something of the soul essence behind the everyday personality of the beloved. One glimpses that 'otherness' and the loved one feels enhanced by that vision. The lover is seeing us and responding to us in a way no one perhaps has done before, and we become radiant. The trouble is that we become dependent upon the vision of our lover. He sees me as more beautiful or clever, but what happens when he turns his eyes away and looks at another? Where am I then?

We meet someone and for a while they open our heart and love pours in. Once we have felt it open, no one can shut it again, unless we allow it to shut. Don't make the mistake of thinking your lovers have the key – that you must beg for it. Yours is the key, a golden key, and you have it in your hands forever.

* * *

Perhaps I was in too much of a rush to get into the next stage of the story. We don't give much time to these more delicate and sensitive areas of our life. We think of them as growing pains or puppy love, but the way I wrote it is the way I remember it. Not feeling particularly hurt or crushed, so much as finding myself taken unawares by this incredible inner feeling I couldn't put a name to. Having it named for me in that way almost killed it stone dead. Or rather it turned it into something secret which couldn't be shared or spoken of. Yes A.Z., I suppose you are right. I became ashamed.

Maybe we too readily accept everyone else's evaluation of our feelings as something trivial to be quickly forgotten. It is odd, too, how we tend to rush away from moments of pain or difficulty in our lives, getting caught up in other excitements, being bright and getting on with life. Yet it is these experiences that we unwittingly hold on to the most, and unconsciously they seem to accumulate into a dark cloud which comes back to haunt us in the wee small hours. But when we have one of those timeless moments of joy, it seems our minds cannot hold it, and we believe it is gone forever.

It is only now, at this much later stage of my life, that I am realising that we do have the power to choose. If in the small hours of the night we lie awake and nothing but gloom seems to surround us, we don't have to succumb. We can use the power of our mind to create a place of sunlight and happiness, by recapturing or building up in our inner world a scene where we once touched joy, and know that it is as real and true as any of the nightmares which we have allowed to take hold. Then, after we have visualised that place, we can soak up its energies – the wind, the waves, the leaves of grass, the healing warmth of the sun.

This will open the way to more of the positive, creative inflow. Then change will slowly but surely begin to take place in our lives. For most of my life I have accepted the ill health, the chaos and bad luck that life seemed to throw at us, as real and inevitable. Yes, one could face these things in the outer world with a kind of courage and do what one could to change them there, but I never understood that I had the power to change my inner world through creative imagination, or that this could positively affect the outer world. Imagination is a tool of the creator: the image arises in the artist's mind and the form follows, manifesting in the solid world. Yet both image (what we call imagination) and form are real.

ARTIST'S LIFE

In September of the year I became fifteen, a group of us from the Junior Department were literally about to step through a new door: the portals of Sheffield's College of Arts and Crafts. We gathered in the street and were joined by several other new recruits, mostly older than us, who had arrived, bedecked with striped art college scarves and a clutch of qualifications, from the city's grammar schools. There was still no Art College building as such, but these premises, at the corner of Arundel Street and Norfolk Street, were much more like the real thing, as the top floor was to all intents and purposes an atelier. The life-rooms, painting and design studios had roof lights and sloping windows, which looked out on the panorama of the city and down on the bustling streets below.

This exhilarating new environment, this sense of life expanding, progressing, climbing upwards, the anticipation of all that might lie ahead, was tempered by a few secret adolescent anxieties. We probably clutched our fears to ourselves not wanting to look foolish, but in confessional whispers we discovered that there was a common nightmare all we innocents shared. How were we going to cope with our first life class?

The naked human body was one of society's greatest taboos in those days. We'd hardly broached the 1950's, and it strikes me now that this first life class could well count as one of those rites of passage into adulthood, an initiation into the Society of the Arts. To the world at large this was the one thing which marked the dividing line between normal, respectable citizens, and those licentious, weird and dangerous artists who sat in a circle gawping at women with no clothes on. All society's fears and fantasies about sex were projected upon the scene. There was a shifting of feet and a tittering when the subject came up: 'Would young female students be impossibly embarrassed?' 'Would they be set upon and stripped by the young male students unable to contain their lust?' 'How would the young men manage to keep their drawing boards resting on their laps?' 'Would there be orgies at the drop of a hat?' Such were the fantasies of the populace! Strangely no one said 'I wonder how you will cope with drawing such an interesting and complex subject?'

I don't think even we had that in mind as a priority when we settled ourselves for our first encounter with the nude. Yet, from the moment the model disrobed and the pose was set, an extraordinary hush and calm descended upon the class. And it was always like this. There is something about the human body which calls out a marvelling and a reverence and an appetite – a desire – to recreate that marvellousness, excitement, wonder on the white sheet of paper. Standing at your easel, the air becomes charged with creative tension. Models young and old, enormous or petite, dignified or vulgar, ugly or beautiful are both gobbled up *and* clinically observed. The detachment of the surgeon and the sensual delight of the lover are combined, synthesised and transcended in the creative act. We celebrated the human form and perspired in our efforts to capture our vision. But almost always our struggles to draw a hand with just the right emphasis of pressure upon a hip, or buttock upon the chair, left us feeling disappointed and frustrated.

Feelings were even more inadequate when a tutor would sit down beside us, pick up our drawing board and make a drawing beside our own that left us feeling breathless and awe-struck. One of our drawing masters, a man every inch the popular image of the artist of the day: aquiline nose, goatee beard, and on occasion sporting a silk-lined cloak and silver-topped swordstick, would dazzle us by beginning his demonstration-drawing with the pencil in his left hand.

Starting at the right foot, he would proceed with a beautiful sinuous line which would flow across the paper, bringing to life the character of the model as he worked upwards to the top of the head. Whereupon he would transfer the pencil to his right hand, and complete the drawing to his satisfaction and our delight by the exact placing of the left foot, with perfect balance and proportion. He had been a student of Augustus John and his drawings were every bit as masterly. As a teacher he inspired and conveyed by example, a love, not only of drawing, but of the grandeur of the Italian Renaissance, painting, sculpture and architecture, to several generations of students. I am intensely proud, as well as unbelieving still, to have been given his 'prize for drawing' for a sketch I made of a young woman, whilst on my first trip to France when I was eighteen.

The 'Augustus John' thing provided us with an image to identify with, for a time. This flamboyant painter was legendary for his unconventional, bohemian lifestyle: living with gypsies, having a series of wives and mistresses and innumerable children. His paintings were full of vivacity and colour and swirling energy. Pinks, reds, ochres, oranges and yellows were his palette, and after the austerities of the war, this liberation of flowing skirts and hair and the insinuations of free love was reason for wanting to imitate his style.

One of the students in our year, Michael John Corbidge, had a great talent in draughtsmanship, and a lot of bravado. Enough to carry him on a painting scholarship to the Slade School in London a year before the rest of us. He had been so smitten with Augustus and his romantic lifestyle, that soon after he arrived and found himself surrounded by glamorous but naive young girl students, he set about collecting a harem about him. He dyed his hair and moustache, donned some outrageous bohemian clothes and called himself Michael John. They fell for the tale, at least for a while, that he was one of Augustus' brood of illegitimate children and had inherited some of his genius.

Dressing up and posing was fun when all around was drab conformity. The streets of Sheffield in the rush hour for some years after the war could easily have been taken for Moscow, with men in overalls or navy working clothes, and women in uniform, utility, knee-length skirts and head-scarves. Art students were allowed and expected to be unconventional and we stepped into our roles with great enthusiasm, using our ingenuity and creativity. I once walked alone, from the bottom of The Moor at one end of town to Fitzallen Square at the other, bare footed, swirling a long gathered skirt made from a heavy, woven Victorian cover, and a fringed, black lace shawl which I'd bought in Portobello Road on a trip to London! On my head was a straw boater with a red ribbon which I'd found among some old clothes in the wardrobe, and round my waist, a large dog-collar with brass studs. The cheek, bravado or courage it took to do that, when every head turned to stare and every mouth gaped open, either in verbal or unspoken comment as I passed by, can't be imagined today when anything goes.

Student Rag Day was another opportunity to be outrageous, but this time sanctioned by a good cause. The Art College vied with the University for the best and most original ideas for floats. One year a group of art students bedecked themselves as lepers with twisted limbs and crutches and eaten-into faces. They were so realistic that they had half the population of Sheffield running from them in panic.

The boat race was the highlight of the day: a bizarre event in the extreme, in which the most unlikely crews in the most fantastic craft set sail. It culminated at the weir at Lady's Bridge. The river Don in those days was so polluted that streams of livid colours, sickening purples and ochres and blues, poured into it at that point, mingling with stinking browns and greys, bubbling gasses and hissing steams. I wouldn't have gone into that water in reality, for a king's ransom, but this turgid river became another of the features of my dream-life for decades afterwards. I would find myself swimming upstream, battling against its current night after night, only to awake the next morning feeling poisoned and debilitated. I can only rejoice when I see the Don today, cleaned up to such an extent that willow trees and wild flowers, and even nesting birds, have colonised the once lethal banks.

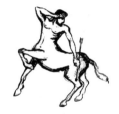

A BLOOMING BUNCH

Whatever influence our family and home background had on us in the past was diminishing now, as we became gathered as a body, into a group relationship. Three days a week there were evening classes, which meant having a bite to eat in town rather than returning home for tea, so that we were spending most of our time together and our contact with home and local friends was growing fainter. A wonderful comradeship and friendship began to develop in which we found ourselves explorers, going off on our own or in pairs, with sketch book and colours into unknown territory. Backstreets of old Sheffield reminiscent of Dickensian times were uncovered. We seemed to sniff out idiosyncratic alleyways, and characterful old streets and houses which few people knew about.

It was the twisted chimneys, uneven pathways of old York stone, wrought-iron lamps suspended between alley walls creating an interplay of fleeting light and shade, or eerie bomb-ruined churches with ragwort and rosebay willowherb sprouting from the rubble, that were the subjects of our work. With this booty carefully captured in our sketch books we would return to base – to the group – and eventually our best efforts would be selected and thrown into the common pool, and pinned up for one of the regular class sketch-club exhibitions. There was a constant exchange of energies going on – individual exploration and discoveries being fed back into the pool, and then some sort of evaluation of our process as we compared each other's compositions and saw how others had interpreted their experiences.

It was at some point during these first years that a large old building, an ex-Bluecoat School, was found for the Art College to occupy, and we moved into the leafy suburbs. At last we had space, we had grounds and marble staircases, a new status and classical proportions. Moreover, we had a dining room and proper catering instead of the two gas rings and sandwiches we had been used to, *and* we had a magnificent common room.

Our real focal point, however, rapidly became centred back in town, in an accommodating café in Norfolk Street, which we dubbed with great originality, 'The Norfolk Caff'. Accommodating, in that it allowed us to sit for hours with just one cup of coffee, or at the most a Welsh rarebit and tea and talk of 'Art' night after night, and year in year out. More was accomplished here through these long philosophising conversations than ever there was in the august halls of our new college. This was our own steamy atmosphere where our heroes, our masters, the lights that inspired us, were discussed endlessly. Artists of the Paris scene, Soutine, Chagall, Rouault, as well as Picasso, Matisse and Braque, were conjured up until they became real to us as teachers. Having such paintings constantly before us, even if only through the reproductions in books, gave us an awareness of light and colour and composition in the every day world around us that hadn't existed before. Walking the old familiar streets of town of an evening we saw Van Gogh's stars reflected in pools of rain water, or Soutine's characters standing at street corners, faces transformed by a combination of our imagination and the lurid red and amber traffic lights. Not only did we have our passions awakened for the visual arts, but we developed avid appetites for literature, and read and discussed the Russian and English writers. Again, the French influence was strong. Sartre, Camus, Simone de Beauvoir, all those writers and philosophers involved in the existentialist movement. The image of the singer Juliette Greco, with her straight black hair, white face and black beret, performing in the left bank cafés of Paris, added an air of dangerous glamour. In fact, the all-black garb, tragic faces and cigarette smoke soon became our new fashion, ousting poor old Augustus John.

Not only did we meet in smoke filled cafés, but there was another side to our activities. The Peak District, before the ubiquitous ownership of cars, was a solitary wilderness. Walking for miles across the moorland, the comrades were inseparable too. We developed a taste for rock climbing on the glacial edges of Stanedge and Burbage. Became speleologists and delved, crawled and wriggled through the underground passages of Giant's Hole and other local potholes. We slept all together in wet tents, steaming and mud-soaked, bonded in warm friendship.

At college we were fed with an array of techniques and skills, materials and media, and our first three years were spent imbibing a rich diet of experiences and possibilities. We were offered charcoal and pastel, goose-quill pens and reed pens, oils, gouache, dyes and enamels, and many more tools of the trade to try. We painted and designed, sculpted in clay and stone, we threw pots and we etched. We were taught lithography, letter cutting, silver work and jewellery, furniture design and making, dress design, weaving and much, much more.

We were instructed in the disciplines of anatomy and architecture, the science of perspective and the history of art, and at the end of three years we would take the important Intermediate Exam. Those of us who passed this milestone would go on to specialise for the next two years in one medium or craft, whichever we felt most drawn to out of the many areas we had experimented with in those first years.

Deciding whether to become painters or sculptors seemed to be the only real options to consider for the comrades of that Norfolk Caff hot-house. Our sights were already set on 'making it into the big time' via one of the top London postgraduate colleges: Royal College, Slade School of Fine Art, or perhaps the Royal Academy if we couldn't manage one of the other two. We didn't see it as egotistic ambition, but as a serious goal to aim at. For serious we were about fashioning ourselves into true artists.

Student fashions, role playing and the camaraderie of the group are all part of the rewards of art school life, and the development of our skills and gifts goes hand in hand with the fun. But the student artist is in the process of becoming an adult artist, and this deepening of understanding of purpose needs to take place also, if one is to sustain a lifetime of dedication to art. This understanding can only grow at the pace of the individual, and it can't be taught. It will also be a personal journey of discovery, and there will be a different journey of creative unfoldment for each one.

It seems to me now, that the business of the painter or sculptor is above all about communication and about developing the senses. Particularly the development of the faculty of vision. As you learn to draw there is a growing co-ordination of hand and eye. Looking deeper and harder you begin to see in a way that brings you closer into relationship with the object of that looking. And it is not too far fetched to say that the act of looking becomes an act of love. The humblest object will begin to reveal itself to you as your gaze penetrates and opens up its secrets. I found myself often being taken unawares in those days. Perhaps walking along some nondescript street of soot-blackened brick houses and finding myself stopped beside a wall I had passed a hundred times before. My eyes became engaged by the texture and pattern of a few bricks, seeing for the first time glints of pearly green, apricot, bronze or purple, yellow, gold or silver among the familiar terracotta and grey which I had superficially assumed.

I remember reading some years later Aldous Huxley's account of his experiments with the new drug Mescaline, forerunner of LSD, in his book *The Doors of Perception*. He describes how someone placed a small vase with a single iris on his table, and how the drug's effect on the mind opened to him this wonderful, spiritual experience of living colour, of an intensity far beyond natural eyesight, and one which flowed on and on timelessly – out of time. But I think this intensity, this touching of a heightened reality, can be there without resorting to a drug. Maybe the engagement of an artist with a flower or a landscape, or whatever, can become at times more like a meditation, and that heightened state of consciousness can be available to anyone who will learn to be still and receptive.

The problem arises when the person experiencing the vision attempts to capture something of it on the page. How to communicate through pigment the wonder and beauty of the vision. Those artists who have achieved the near miracle in the past are our masters, and sometimes the gap between the vision and the personal result is too much to bear. Yet perhaps we need these lights before us to inspire and encourage us. We need others who have trod upon mountain tops and discovered ways to weave visions out of clay, miracles from thin air.

* * *

Within the warm embrace of the group, more and more now, pair relationships were forming. Feelings of attraction, sometimes to the most unlikely people, were born. There were flirtations, dalliances, setting out of stalls. At last two people would decide to settle for one another, and it seemed that after some amorous adventures on my part in one or two other directions, Brian Fielding and I would at last become a couple.

Unlike me, although we shared a Piscean birthday, Brian had an intense, energetic yet practical approach to life. He was ardent in his passions whether for football (he was born within spitting distance of Sheffield Wednesday's ground) art, or personal feelings. He believed in and supported me as an artist, and loved me as a woman. Our shared experiences, our delight in nature, our struggles to express ourselves in paint or clay, our conversations, our intimacies, became the precious strands of a cloth which we wove together. Bit by bit its fabric enfolded us, our relationship deepened, and our artistic sensitivities developed. The abstract painter John Hoyland, one of the major figures on the contemporary British Art scene from the sixties onwards, was a young student with me in the Junior Art School days. He was also one of the group who huddled among the teacups and smoke discussing 'Art' in that Norfolk Street Café. Writing in an obituary (*The Independent, The Daily Telegraph*) after Brian's death in 1987 about their close lifelong friendship, he speaks of the impact it had on their early artistic development. He comments: 'Brian was wise and funny, but most of all he was subtle ... inspirational to his students ... aware of every aspect of ART and its underlying philosophies.' He remembers walking the streets of Sheffield together as students, evoking impressions of their heroes,

Rouault and Van Gogh. What *I* remembered, however, were the long days we spent together in the countryside absorbing and being absorbed into the vast spaces and the bleak and rugged dramas of the Peak.

I remember vividly the winter's day Brian and I walked through sleet and hailstones in a kind of awed silence along the Roman causeway by Redmires. This took us on to the weirdly shaped outcrop of rocks above Stanedge which have been blasted into prehistoric monster shapes, trolls and crouching gnomes, by the frost and wind. The skies were a glowering leaden grey, heavy with snow, and the wind was biting and blowing directly into our faces. We were kept going by our sheer amusement as every so often an even more incredible troll would lunge at us out of the swirling mist and sleet. Another time we had gone on a hot spring day to the ramparts of Carl's Wark, a kind of fortress of rock standing out grimly and majestically against the sky. As we walked through heather along gritty sheep tracks and through the moorland monochromes of browns and greys, we became aware of 'presence'. Faint spiritual voices of long departed people. The contours of the landscape had evoked not only another time, but another place, a desert kingdom, a rocky temple complex. We were catching sounds and scenes of ancient Babylon. It was weird and eerie and we didn't have the vocabulary to express what we were sensing to one another. Later we began persuading each other that our imagination had got the better of us.

On our many ramblings together we had sharp eyes for tiny things, and were forever picking up fragments of root, fungus, fragile eggshells, quartz crystals. Finding skulls, bones, ram's horns in the melting snow, casualties of the winter just gone by. A piece of weathered stone like a human torso or forms even more fantastic would be spotted like trophies for the collection, and borne back in triumph. It was a landscape of ancient presences and earth energies as well as the remains of last year's dead sheep. We came upon half hidden megaliths and stone circles, long barrows and menhirs and once, a hermit's cave with a crude crucifix carved on the wall. These we drew or painted on the spot and made pictures which seemed to capture the magical quality that went with us on these walks.

A.Z. FIFTH COMMENTARY

I asked Astrazzurra if he would like to comment. 'I am sorry,' I told him, 'but I seem to have left you quite an area to cover…'

Yes. I am running my mind over those years. This is what I see. You are young and opening out to many new things. All is at your feet – all is to come – like a tide rushing in. Such delights, new experiences, new growth; establishing your roots in the soil of your culture; bedding down in the richness of that soil. Everywhere around you is golden promise.

You have the city, literally, at your feet, and below you is bustle and commerce, dirt, sweat and heat. It is also a blackened city with its fiery furnaces glowing and slag-heaps scarring the landscapes and poisoning the soil. Rivers polluted, smog and gas, sulphur and acid rain eating into the fabric, damaging buildings and plants alike. All around is devastation as well as triumph and achievement.

This is your cultural heritage: a rich soil and an exhausted land, both at the same time. Riches and ruin together. You are suffering from this now; even now. You have taken into yourself the atmosphere of poison, both of the home, which you told about earlier, and of the city. You were aware of it and felt it keenly. You wanted to do something to aid the city, to bring some green leaves and fresh air into it. A city needs to breathe from the heart. It needs a healthy Heart Chakra. The element associated with the Heart Chakra is AIR, and GREENNESS is its colour.

Many of you were drawn to the open countryside around the city. The beautiful landscape of Derbyshire and the Peak District was somewhere for students and citizens alike to delight in and escape to. By going out and filling your lungs with the air and drawing deeply on the beauty that your senses perceived, you brought that back with you and integrated it into your life and art. Some of you went into it and immersed yourselves into it even more deeply by contacting the earth in the underground caves and tunnels, and climbing with hands and feet, fingernails and toes, up the rocky faces of glacial edges. Feeling the touch of limestone and grit-stone, lichen and moss.

You immersed yourselves in the seasons: the snows of winter and the dryness and heat of summer, the damp mouldering richness of autumn and the quickening of the spring. All this you breathed into yourselves as you breathed out the enervated air and smokiness of the city, releasing pollution from your auras. As you cleansed and refreshed yourselves, you created an exchange of energies which helped to cleanse the city's aura also, until at last the consciousness of the people was raised enough to bring about an influence which resulted in a clean-air policy, and the soot and grime was washed away.

Over all of this Vulcan watched from his position high over the city.[*] Vulcan is one of the Gods and in his heart great matters are being pondered. He is an archetype of great transformative power. Flame and fire. The Fire of the Gods triumphant and splendid.

He dwells in the hearts of men and will bring triumph at last over the powers of evil and darkness, pollution and sickness. He will triumph. I speak of 'He' but this is just an image. What I speak of is an energy of high frequency and form. Call him a God: he is a powerful force that will serve you well.

He comes on wings of Flame and Light to ensure victory for you over the powers of darkness embedded in matter. He will lift you up and help raise you to the state of the immortals. He surmounts the city and sees what goes on down through the ages. He sees the struggles and the hardship, he has also seen the greed and the cunning and the lack of love. He has seen people whose desire for riches was so strong that they had no care or feeling for who or what they exploited in the process of making money.

Then the joy of life was killed off; the sparkle of the water, the clarity of the air was sucked away in the race for wealth. So the real wealth was stolen. The gifts that were bestowed by God in the beginning were despoiled as substances were extracted. Coal, metal, oxygen, health, energy, and well-being were eaten up, and the ravaged substances, sucked dry of their virtue, were spat out to poison the earth. When such things are grabbed in this way without love or respect, and no reparation is made, then great wounds are caused and sickness results. Sickness of the earth and the people.

The God called Vulcan watched this take place and grieved for you all. His heart was afire with his love for you. As he looked down he sought those spirits whom he could work with – young and old – fashioners and creators – not of wealth in the material sense, but wealth in love and spirit. Those in whom beauty was awakening and those who

---

[*] There is a statue of Vulcan on top of Sheffield Town Hall.

responded to beauty and wished to create more. He sent you his blessings as he is blessing you now.

Many of you have been inspired to restore and heal your city. Some of you in small, quiet, secret ways, and some of you in louder and more public ways. When you yourself strove to uplift the depleted energies of the place in your unconscious night journeys, Vulcan saw this. He blessed his artists and his craftsmen and women. Parts of the city are now greatly improved with clean buildings, spaces and trees, but there is much more still to do.

There is further to go: far more is happening than you can be aware of, and more than you ever dreamed of. A transformation will take place in the near future which will astound you, and you will have direct conscious experience of it soon. Deep down a regeneration is about to occur in the landscape. Slumbering roots will awaken, lambs will jump for joy and a great harvest will be gathered in. There is a new understanding about to be born.

Those of you who have been called to be healers, imaginers, dreamers and creators, will be empowered to bring about this regeneration. You will be co-creators and workers for the Light as you link together and work on the astral plane. I have spoken to you before about the astral planes and how our desires and longings are communicated and transmitted through that element, and of our links with you there. There have already been communications with you at a deep and, for the most part, unconscious level.

In certain levels of sleep we contact you, and many of the inspirations that you wake with are occasioned by our contact. You are learning while you sleep. We implant ideas into your mind, when you are ready and have given your consent to such teaching within your soul. In the sleep state there is better access to you at a level where you yourselves are freer from some of the old ways of understanding – the mind-sets that you occupy in the wakeful state. And so ideas are set going and we can open up possibilities for you, visions and vistas of other dimensions which you might not consider in everyday life.

Avenues of approach are suggested and help is also given when you request it of us. Many of the so called chance encounters or coincidences in life come about because lines of energy are drawn together here on our planes, so that significant meetings may occur. So be conscious and aware of what you ask for. It might well be given you.

FOUR

ODE

We are the music makers,
And we are the dreamers of dreams,
Wandering by lone sea-breakers,
And sitting by desolate streams;
World-losers and world-forsakers,
On whom the pale moon gleams:
Yet we are the movers and shakers
Of the world for ever, it seems.

With wonderful deathless ditties
We build up the world's great cities,
And out of a fabulous story
We fashion an empire's glory:
One man with a dream, at pleasure,
Shall go forth and conquer a crown;
And three with a new song's measure
Can trample a kingdom down.

We, in the ages lying
In the buried past of the earth,
Built Nineveh with our singing,
And Babel itself with our mirth;
And o'erthrew them with prophesying
To the old of the new world's worth;
For each age is a dream that is dying,
Or one that is coming to birth.

A. W. E. O'Shaughnessy 1844-1881

PEAKS CROWNS CAPITALS

Reflecting on some of the things A.Z. has been saying in the earlier chapters on childhood times – drawing my attention to the affinity children have with nature and our need to be nurtured by Mother Earth – it seems regrettable that the student years I am now covering will take me further into the conglomerations of concrete, tarmac, traffic and congestion of Europe's great cities. I can feel now, with the luxury of retrospection, how urgent is the necessity of allowing children to awaken their souls to the deep currents of instinctual knowing. This can be imparted through contact with the energy of flowing water and trees, the massiveness of mountains, the vastness of deserts, or from contact with animal instinctual wisdom. These are rarely, if ever, given the importance they should have in our so-called education systems. In fact, time devoted to just 'being' and open receptiveness, as opposed to actively cramming our heads with facts, has been regarded as time-wasting, idleness, drifting and dreaming. Yet the soul as well as the body thrives on this nourishment because it feeds our imagination and our creative powers.

This is not to deny, however, that there is a spiritual urge in mankind to build and to create cities. Architecture is a sacred calling, and has been from the earliest periods of mankind's history and cultural development. We have looked upwards to the stars and been inspired to express the cosmic grandeur of design, pattern and order we have somehow discerned in the heavens. We have felt our dependency and our interrelatedness with the powerful rhythms of the cycles of the seasons, which the movement of the planets, the rising and setting of the sun, and waxing and waning of the moon initiate.

Across the world, from age to age, temples have been constructed in alignment with celestial bodies. The great stone circles of Stonehenge or Avebury, the sublime classical proportions of the Acropolis, are all earthly representations of our sense of the sacred. These constructions were the Houses of the Gods and were located on mountains or in other numinous places where there was already, before anyone had placed one pebble upon another, a sense of awe and mystery associated with Divine habitation.

Temples were places set apart and approached with reverence, but gradually human settlements would be built around these sacred sites. Priests and astronomers had to be housed, and next in hierarchical importance were the architects, musicians and artists. Systems of healing evolved, and temples of the healing arts were created where initiates could be trained and the sick could be brought in. Then came settlements for artisans, markets, storage for produce, and as all this had to be protected from marauders, police forces and armies were formed. Thus, cities came into being, evolving from an original pattern which proceeded from a heavenly ordering – man reaching upwards, *aspiring* to recreate his vision of the celestial world here on Earth, and the heavens reaching down, *inspiring* man's creations.

We may well have lost touch with the original sense of sacredness which lay behind the emergence of cities, and forgotten or be ignorant of the geometry of the heavens on which they were based. Yet something of this lives on in the collective unconscious mind and emerges from time to time in our dreams.

Just as I felt drawn back to my roots by the voice of nature, so there was also a counter force drawing me towards civilisation – if I can use that word in its original meaning. For it means just that. Its root is from the Latin *civilitas* meaning 'civilize', through *civitas* or 'city'. I believe that Civilisation is again one of the archetypal forces stemming from Divine Order, this time expressed through Geometry and Number, and that it is a power at work throughout the created Universe. The golden mean ratio which Pythagoras and Plato demonstrated, and on whose proportions the Parthenon was constructed, is the very same principle which governs the growth patterns of shells and many flowers: nautilus shells and sunflowers being prime examples. But just as the sunflower is unconscious of the power which guides its form and growth, I too was unconscious of the forces at work behind the scenes in my life.

At this juncture it is possible to detect strands and themes running through the last ten years in a way that wasn't possible at the time. Between the ages of fifteen and twenty-five many physical and psychological changes take place. It is no wonder that for most of us our full attention is on the outer world. The inner world of *in*tuition, of psychic sensing – ways of perceiving not dependant on the physical senses, is sadly neglected.

There may have been many strange dreams during those years, and some of them recurring, repeating a theme time and again. Yet I didn't have the insight or understanding to pause and listen to the messages they were trying to give me. No one around me, none of the books I had read, up until that point, gave any indication of the important part our unconscious mind plays in warning us when we are becoming out of balance with our true selves. Nor of the rich storehouse of collective and personal mythology the unconscious makes available to us, and how we can dip into and replenish ourselves from it. The unconscious mind was dismissed in the same way that nature was dismissed.

Yet dreams there were, and over and again I would dream that I was present in some magnificent city of spacious squares with fountains playing, majestic buildings with classical porticoes, ascending flights of steps, symmetrically placed, which led to the entrance of an awe-inspiring edifice. Often I would be viewing all this from a great height, suspended in the air, or perched on some high turret or Gothic spire from where there was a clear sense of the mandala-like plan, the symmetrical and harmonious design of the unknown city below. I would wake from these dreams feeling that I had somehow been transported during the night and been returned to everyday life with a feeling of inspiration and renewal.

But there were other dreams, increasingly nightmarish, where I was climbing up sheer faces of rock with toe and finger-holds growing ever more minimal until they almost disappeared. As the rock face grew almost vertical, it became smoother and smoother, and the ground an impossible, sickening, vertigo-inducing distance away. Then I would wake in the morning sweating and knotted up with tension, only to find I had over-slept and had to rush to college without breakfast yet again. It was simpler to brush these off as 'only dreams', rather than spend precious time seriously trying to understand what they were attempting to tell me.

As I scan that ten year period again, three key words seem to spring out: Peaks, Crowns and Capitals. Whatever it was that had initially induced me to take up the sport of climbing, something must have touched an inner urge unconsciously waiting to express itself. I don't assume I was alone; it is likely that I was tapping into a fairly common experience – the urge to pit oneself against 'The Mountain' – whatever that mountain might signify individually. For some it may symbolise the stronghold of the gods, the footstool of the sky, while for others it represents nature in its rawest, most awesome aspect, and the great challenge which he or she, insignificant speck, impulsively feels the need to conquer. Yet again, for some it might symbolise climbing the promotional ladder, a rise in pay or a seat on the board. For others it will be the achievement of fame and fortune. Whatever its personal significance, climbing the mountain can be seen as a reflection of the ego's developmental process: consciousness of 'self', the individual, testing out the limits of that self, and having that achievement recognised, rewarded or praised. And the awards or scholarships – these glittering prizes, these crowns of glory – these are what we strive for in the hope that public acknowledgement will affirm our self-worth.

The drive which propels us towards a personal goal, some obstacle to overcome, victory to achieve, summit to conquer, is an evolutionary energy forging qualities of courage, will and fortitude which might never have been developed without the ego-urge. Yet as we know, egos can get out of hand. Egos are all very well and an important stage in our development, but most of us get stuck there when we could be moving on into something more interesting, and far more useful. If we can only think of the 'self' with a small 's', as being on a journey towards the Self with a capital 'S', the Higher Self, then there can come a renewed vigour and enthusiasm, and also a greater meaning to life as we begin to glimpse the possibilities of true freedom which that new vision holds out for us. It may well be that the thrust which stirred our egos to climb to the mountain top is the very same energy which will carry us beyond the ego and into a new and undreamed of world of empowerment and freedom. A world unfettered by selfish interest and the limitations it imposes.

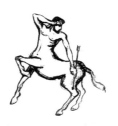

TRAVELLING SCHOLARS

I had opted to specialise in sculpture. It was no well thought out rational decision, but one prompted mainly by feeling. It had been the touch and smell of the materials and the actual sense of bodily engagement with one's creation – the three-dimensionality of it, if I can put it that way. The joy of working with my hands, the earthiness of the mediums of expression – clay, stone, wood, metal – as well as the relationship of form to space which had seduced me. Tactile sense, kinaesthetic sense, are terms I learned much later. They may express it better. But as I think I have said before, I didn't easily express myself in words in those days in spite of the mass of literature I had read. I seemed to understand things deeply but intuitively, not intellectually.

Brian had opted for painting and we found ourselves, for the next two years, working apart. The three-dimensional studios: pottery, carving, silversmithing, and so on, were still in downtown basements and cellars, while all the other activities were in the new college building in the suburbs. Towards the end of our last year, we simultaneously managed to achieve the award of a small travelling scholarship to Europe, and were actually going to be paid for doing something exciting and pleasurable. Thus we set off for the Continent via London, approaching the whole adventure as a feast laid out before us. With a bit of cash we had saved by foregoing a midday meal for a couple of terms, we made the adventure stretch out several weeks longer than our award money allowed.

After saturating ourselves with the treasures of the British Museum and the galleries of London, we departed, packs on backs, to hitch-hike to Paris. We rented, in true Bohemian style, a garret in Monte Martre. We bought bottles of wine and drank them at the foot of the Sacré Coeur, and immediately became intoxicated, not so much by the alcohol as by the heady atmosphere of the city. It was as though, sitting there on the steps of this great cathedral towering above us on the hill, white in the moonlight, drinking our wine straight from the bottle, we were honouring the spirit of artistic and cultural France. There was a sense also of paradox. Everything strange and new. The sounds, the lights, the outdoor festiveness and gaiety of the street-life, so different from the post-war greyness of London. Yet we felt, at the same time, that we had come home. Paris welcomed and understood two would-be members of the international brotherhood of artists.

We were eager to immerse ourselves in that atmosphere. The smells – utterly foreign and enticing – Gauloises, garlic, Gallic drains. Aromas of fresh bread, patisserie, and coffee wafting from pavement cafés; strange and delicious savours, that made us long to sample this extraordinary menu. Yet, like hungry beggars, we contented ourselves with watching others partake of the feast, and ate only cheese and bread sans butter, so that we could spend our money on drawing materials and visiting the Louvre and the Orangerie where the wonderful canvases of Cézanne and Matisse were hung. We dropped in on every little exhibition. We filled our sketchbooks and notebooks with detailed studies from museums, made quick impressions of people on riverbanks, in parks or pavement cafés. We crammed in as much as we could of the life and the history all around us.

Unable to afford the price of the bus or Metro, we walked Paris from end to end, becoming hungrier and thinner. All my travels during those ten years seem to be scored on my psyche in terms of aching legs and a perpetual hunger for the wonderful food that others seemed to be constantly enjoying, but that I was not allowed. Maybe we had taken too seriously the myth of the starving artist, and were working on the assumption that hunger was one of the requirements of genius. The comforts of life were decidedly sacrificed in the name of our art, for we slept at night in cheap and squalid beds, if we slept in beds at all, and walked the streets by day until our legs threatened to drop off. But what did that matter if we had encountered Mona Lisa or the Venus de Milo, or had rested by the feet of a striding pharaoh in an empty and silent gallery examining his toenails at leisure.

The Louvre had been particularly crowded around those two renowned works of art, and I had felt rather impatient with the sheep-like mentality of the tourists who always thronged around a painting with a reputation. But when, after browsing through side galleries for a while, I happened upon the Venus de Milo unawares, I was mindblown by the sheer presence and beauty of that fragmented female. The weathered texture of the stone draperies clinging to her strong and graceful legs, the confidence and poise of her demeanour, told me I was in the presence of a goddess indeed, and I apologised to her creator for being unkind about her crowd of worshippers. If she had been merely perfect, her upper limbs complete, her marble complexion polished, her waist a little more slender or the folds of her gown silken and seductive, I would have passed her by. But it seemed that nature had collaborated with the sculptor's chisel, and had interacted in the creative process. Those same elemental forces which sculpt mountains and ravines – the wind, the waves, the sun, the rain – had helped to form those draperies, that texture of hair and skin, and by so doing had raised her above the human ideal of erotic love goddess. They had united in this eternal woman: forces earthy, sexual and divine.

Hoping to avoid the crowd once more, I wandered into the Egyptian Gallery. There was still a fair number of people milling around and I was inwardly sighing and wishing that I could have the gallery to myself. I felt drawn to the Egyptian sculptures, and wanted to commune with them in peace. Also my legs and feet were aching and I couldn't see anywhere to perch. I went further and deeper into the long gallery, until I came to a tall standing figure of a pharaoh. He was on a plinth a few inches high and, hoping no one would notice, I sat down on the base of the statue by his feet. It felt at once restful and companionable. I began to examine his feet. The room had gone very quiet suddenly and I looked up, realising that everyone had mysteriously dispersed. As if my wishes had been answered, I had the enormous gallery to myself.

I became passionately interested in those toes and beautifully carved nails. I had been told by my tutor that sculptors in those days took the greatest care to give attention to every detail, even where, in some cases, the figure would have been covered with a fine layer of gesso and then had colour applied to the surface, so no one would have seen the carved detail beneath. In these ancient times, figures which were made to stand in an elevated position with their backs tight against a pediment or a temple wall and only their fronts displayed to the onlooker, had their backs carved with equal care. Maybe this information was given to us in the hope that we would revere the true artist's integrity and not be tempted into slipshod ways. But I was intrigued to find it was true.

I was intently admiring the shape of each individual toe, relieved that I was alone and could scrutinise him at leisure. I let my gaze travel slowly upwards and began to realise what an immensely powerful presence he presented. He was over life-size, standing with one leg forward in the traditional striding manner. I sat quietly for some time, silently observing and admiring. He seemed to be growing more powerful the longer I looked, and I could almost envisage him in the blazing heat and light of his desert kingdom. There seemed to be an energy and light emanating from him, and as I sat there I began to feel uncomfortable. Perhaps it wasn't quite fitting to be counting his toenails in this casual and intimate manner! Yet he seemed to be a beneficent presence. Even so, my discomfort grew as the energy field around him in which I was sitting grew stronger and more tangible. It seemed to be vibrating, even humming.

I got to my feet and moved away, stupidly conscious that I was beginning to feel afraid. It suddenly seemed more than just coincidence that I was still the only human being in such a vast space, when the other galleries, I could hear, in the distance, were full of the sounds of shuffling feet and the voices of visitors. Once again I began accusing myself of letting my imagination get the better of me. It wasn't until some few years later, when I was a student in the sculpture department at the Royal College of Art and we were gathered in a small studio listening to a visiting lecturer, that I discovered there may have been something more than an over-active imagination at work that day when I sat at the pharaoh's feet.

The visiting lecturer was an Egyptologist who had specialised in the sculptures and the working practices of Egyptian artists, and we were rapt in attention as he led us with him, by the force of his narrative, into the dark, narrow passages of the tombs. He was relating how he had first come across one of the standing figures placed in the centre of an inner room. This chamber, he said, was very dark with one small opening for light up in the ceiling. It was cut in such a way that the light from the sun would come in at an angle acting almost like a spotlight. The shaft of light would travel across the floor as the sun travelled the sky, and at one particular point of day, maybe at noon, it would shine directly on top of the pharaoh's crown, lighting it from above with gold. The effect upon the onlooker entering the dark room at that precise moment, was the impression that the figure was striding forwards.

This dramatic piece of information, although it didn't directly relate to my weird experience, was giving me some deeper understanding of the ritualistic meanings and the religious beliefs behind the carved figures. At that time I was pretty ignorant of the history of Egyptian times, and my chief interest in the works of art had been aesthetic. The next piece of news however, did make me sit up. He was talking now about the hierarchical position of the sculptor: the importance of that calling. The training of the sculptors was much like that of the priests. In fact, the place where the sculptors worked – the name they gave to the atelier or studio – was the same that they had for the sacred sanctuary where the priests performed their rites and communed with their gods and goddesses.

Sculptors, just like priests, were initiated as intermediaries between the living pharaoh and the god presence, which the pharaoh represented on Earth. It fell to the sculptor to imbue the spiritual presence, the soul-energy of the pharaoh, into the carved figure representing his human likeness. It was believed that, once the king had died and gone to his celestial kingdom, his presence and his power would remain on Earth, radiating and emanating from the figure which the sculptor had carved and empowered.

None of this knowledge was available to me on that day in the Louvre, however. Only the sense that I had encountered something unnerving and enticing. A vague sense that there were doorways which might open out into unknown and unexplored territories on every side, leading who knows where? But I hadn't the time or inclination to explore further then. There was enough work to be done in that present time, assimilating, digesting and giving expression to new creations and ideas that would come from the stimulus of our latest experiences.

Soon after this excursion abroad the final exams would be upon us, and there would be a feverish preparation of work to be sent off to London as applications for a place at the Slade School of Fine Art or the Royal College. Much to our relief and amazement we received letters from London summoning us to interviews. Out of that original group of twenty-five young and naive students who had climbed the stairs and nervously settled around the model's throne for that first life class five years ago, almost half, a round dozen, were finally rewarded by a place at one of the top London colleges. The intake for the postgraduate colleges was drawn from all over the British Isles and beyond, and according to the law of averages one would suppose that one or two students from each of the art schools around the country would find themselves selected. But, every so often, there seems to be a flowering of talent in one place, and the sun at that time seemed to be shining on the north of England. This year it was Sheffield which produced its blooms, a year or two later it was Leeds, but all of a sudden the soft and sophisticated South had to sit up and take note. Young artists of all kinds, writers, poets, playwrights, musicians, as well as painters and sculptors, were springing up out of the uncultured and barbaric northern lands.

PROMISE

The mountain, it seems, was conquered: we had reached our goal. Yet personally, I was to find that what seemed to be the summit, once you have arrived, soon becomes just a stepping-stone to another peak. Finding a place to live and settling in were the first priorities, but it soon began to sink in that very powerful influences were at work, which would bring about a new phase of learning and growth.

The Royal College was, at that time, housed in the same building as the Victoria and Albert Museum. Except for the sculpture and ceramics departments, which, following the usual form, were relegated to an out of the way piece of land, an ex-Life Guards barracks sandwiched somewhere between the Science Museum and the Natural History Museum. But it was a quick, short step along a pathway between the museums to the V & A and into the painting school where all my friends were situated.

In contrast with the northern provincial Art College, which had been fairly gentle and nurturing, life in that great Victorian imperial complex at South Kensington was inspiring. Imposing museums, colleges, monuments, avenues, all constructed, it seemed, with the purpose of demonstrating the excellence and dominance, both scientific and artistic, of the cultural achievements of the British Empire, made their presence felt. Whether they most inspired awe, scepticism, fear, or hope, I can't judge. It took people in different ways. But simply being in daily contact with those edifices and spaces; the grand avenues leading to Hyde Park; Queen's Gate, Exhibition Road, or the Albert Hall, the Royal College of Music or the V & A itself, one couldn't help absorbing something of their power and influence.

It wasn't necessarily a conscious thing. We strolled with casual nonchalance and equal indifference through galleries lined with treasures from Romanesque or Renaissance Europe or rich silken robes from Imperial China, to have our morning cuppa in the tea rooms of the V & A, or in Joe Lyon's down the road by the South Ken underground. We took for granted that this world, which we were temporarily inhabiting, was ours by right. It was only by night that, as those precious years went by, the spirit of the place began to seep into dreams, imposing an unseen and unacknowledged sense of its awe-fullness upon the sleeper's consciousness. Questionings and self-doubts began to stir about the stated and the unspoken expectations that this world was demanding of us.

On every hand we were surrounded by exemplars. Not only was there the resonance of those imperious buildings bringing its influence to bear, but every day we were having to compare ourselves with brilliant and successful human models. Our tutors were no longer safe 'Sunday painters' who taught for a living and exhibited annually in local shows, but were, on the whole, well known artists of national and international repute. We were lectured to by the celebrities of the time, architects and art historians with household names: Basil Spence, Basil Taylor, Sir Hugh Casson; and visited by artists of great fame: Henry Moore and Jacob Epstein, to name but two. It gradually began to filter through to us that what we were about was the attainment of fame and fortune. That this was to be the goal and the measure of successfully completing the course.

We had been selected because we were thought to have that special ingredient, *promise*. But now we were expected to show signs of fulfilling that promise. There was that expectation, unspoken but nevertheless hanging over us, that much had been invested in us. There was, in addition, that relentless inner drive to create the most excellent, most audacious, most beautiful, shocking, revolutionary, original work of art possible. *And* that someone should recognise it, acclaim it, write about it, and above all, pay us large sums of cash for it. Oh! What dreams, and what depths of disappointment we were setting up for ourselves.

Many of these elements were unconscious at the time, pushed aside because one didn't know how to deal with them. Looking at them again has not been easy. Rather like tunnelling through granite inch by inch, chipping away, retrieving material which was there all along, yet too intangible and shadowy to be grasped, too amorphous to be shaped into words. The fear of facing and acknowledging it earlier, and the belief that I couldn't do so, meant that much creative life-energy was petrified and lost to consciousness because it lay so long in the dark. Yet perhaps then was not the best time for acquiring this degree of self-awareness. One was young and full of optimism about the future. All attention and energy directed outwards: working hard, playing equally hard, taking advantage of everything that London had to offer.

It was a time too of revolution in the art world. The Abstract Expressionists were bursting in upon us with examples of paintings which, at first sight, made me, at least, feel as if the ground had disappeared from under my feet. Radical works which left no subject matter with which to engage emotionally, but relied on the impact of colour, shape and the tension created by their juxtaposition on the surface. They did away with all traces of recognisable image.

Familiarity with abstract art and other vital innovations of the twentieth century had formed part of my education. I considered myself fairly adventurous and certainly no philistine where avant-garde art was concerned, but nevertheless I was about to encounter something so new, so disturbing, that my fragile sense of confidence and security was shattered. Comments by Laurence Alloway, the art critic, at a lecture I attended towards the end of my last year at college, burst in on me like an explosive. Quite intentionally, he set out to demolish our attachments to familiar and dearly loved works of art on which we had been nurtured. Anyone who intended to be a serious artist in the future, he had said, would have to strip themselves of the past and all traditional concepts of figurative art. We were to move into a new world where pure mind clear of romantic trappings, and detachment from 'the known', would enable the artist to create an immediate communication with the viewer through the medium of pure colour and shape.

My own work rose out of deep, intuitive feelings, which demanded to be given form. My understanding of what I wanted to communicate was in a process of slow growth. Only gradually did I begin to experiment with abstraction. One figure I made in about 1957, and which was exhibited in the Royal Academy, was of a young girl on the threshold of puberty, yet grave and old before her time. I had seen such children just after the war, when hoards of Displaced Persons, as they were called, swept hither and thither across Europe. Often, an adolescent whose parents had been killed would be in charge of younger children. The haunted, wraithlike appearance of these child-mothers stirred and moved me. The subjects of my art, the themes and ideas I was trying to express, were attempts to communicate the concerns I had about life.

I gradually developed a more abstract style and bird-like creatures began to make their appearance. I was struggling to express something more ethereal, more spiritual, but finding that the materials that the sculptor has to work with force one to conform to the laws of physical matter. Sculptures, by their very nature, have to stand firmly on the earth, or be fixed securely to another construction, whereas my ideas were leading me into impossibilities. Something in my work was struggling to take flight, and I didn't know how to achieve it within the limitations of the material. I became passionately drawn to the work of Brancusi because he seemed to achieve the miracle I was attempting. His birds soared heavenwards by dint of their polished simplicity. Elegant forms, so reduced to abstraction, that almost no feature of the bird remained, save the essence of 'bird' itself. But my efforts to capture the essence seemed to me to fail dismally.

Looking back on this lecture now I see that the state of mind Alloway was describing was perhaps something like the higher levels of consciousness reached in meditation. Levels which go beyond normal awareness, beyond the level where thought processes recreate mental images and are caught up in the ego's fears and deceptions, and reach a state of communion with what we might call 'the Mind of God'. In fact, some of these artists were much influenced by Buddhism. The vast canvas by Mark Rothko, which graced the meditation room at the United Nations building in New York, is a wonderful example. True creativity, I believe, is always at the leading edge of discovery, pushing known and acceptable boundaries ever further outwards. Originality disturbs the conventionally minded. Most people are looking for something pleasant or romantic to decorate their walls, rather than stretch their minds and challenge them. I was convinced, even then, that creativity is not about staying safely within the known, but is about going into the *unknown*. Yet sitting there with my fellow students I was dismayed by what I was hearing. I wasn't ready for any of this. It was all too soon for me, and I felt my world falling apart. My own work, however much I had experimented with abstraction, had always relied on having a link with a recognisable image, human, animal or organic, and was related to the known world and its traditional links to the past. As I came to the end of my years at the RCA I was beset by doubts, confusions and feelings of failure.

* * *

I received a message from A.Z. at some point during the time I was writing this chapter. It wasn't a direct comment on the text, but ran parallel to it and was given more in the form of a lecture.

A.Z. SIXTH COMMENTARY

'APPEARANCES'

When we, as guides to humanity, approach you, we do so with circumspection and with regard for your integrity. We do not wish to intrude or violate your space in any way. Nor do we wish to impose our thoughts upon your mind, or our views from the perspective of our dimension upon you. We come at your invitation.

At your invitation, when we have made contact and developed a relationship with you, so that you have begun to trust that the being you are meeting is already known and trusted by you, then we can relax the preliminaries and, with your consent, approach you more informally and more frequently. In fact, you Esmé, are often aware that I am with you as you go about your daily tasks. I even appear in the bathroom and we talk as you take a shower. I know, and you know, that you have no sense of being intruded upon. You are at home in your skin as in your outer clothing. You are free from those hang-ups and inhibitions which custom imposes, since you have regained, to some extent, the original innocence of the new born child in regard to your body. This is one of the things you may thank your artist's training for, since it has given you this freedom.

We are also free and have no need of 'outer clothing'. Which doesn't necessarily mean that we go about in naked bodies, but that we have no need to hide anything of ourselves from one another, since there is a knowledge that no one wishes to take advantage in any way of our personal space or integrity, because there is mutual respect. We display our beauty to one another. That inner beauty of the soul is our clothing. We can adopt any costume we wish at any moment, but we clothe ourselves in light and colour. No, better to say, we radiate light and colour and we are free to fashion our countenance as we feel is appropriate or fitting to the occasion.

It is our joy and delight to share our beauty with one another. We open ourselves to joy and love, and this act of sharing mirrors and magnifies the joy and love outwards, creating more and more as it is shared. It

111

sings outwards a melody of sound, enrapturing all who hear it and share in it. The Universe is filled with the sound and the song of our joy in one another.

So thus we approach you. Naked in the sense that we withhold nothing from you. Yet that brightness that we shed as we approach you naked, is – can be – so intense that it is too much for your present eyes to behold, or the ears to hear or the nose, the olfactory sense, to discern the fragrance of it all. We therefore need to step-down its intensity to a level where you can tolerate that 'brightness' of all the senses. That is why it has been common for many of you with psychic vision to 'see' us costumed rather than in our light bodies, and often that clothing that you see will be of a conventional nature. You will tend to see what you expect to see, or what you feel comfortable with. If it has been your custom to think of guides as 'Indian with feathered head-dress' or 'Chinese Sage' or 'Egyptian Priestess', this may be how we will approach you at first, in order not to alarm you. Or, if one of these would be the very guise which would cause an affront, then we will try to find the right approach for you.

Yes Esmé, as you sense, I am moving my comments towards your work as an artist and the message you were trying to put across of how artists today – those who have developed a higher sensitivity towards the spiritual and away from the purely popular and commercial aims in their art – are trying to break down the dependence and resistance which people in general have on their image of physical reality.

Before the last century began you had the Impressionists and the Pointillists, just to take one example, who were attempting to move beyond the limitations of vision. They attempted to use paint to give an impression of the brilliance of colour which they saw all around them when the sunlight draws forth a dance and a dazzle in nature. They did this by flecking and dotting the surface of the painting with an admixture of pigment directly onto the canvas. Always striving to find means to deliver their vision more truly, and finding that the pigments mixed on their pallettes could never quite sing the same note as those colours they saw in the leaves, flowers or water before them, they experimented with mixing elements of primary colour pigment in tiny dots side by side on the surface of the painting, allowing the white of the background to shine through and play its part. Then the viewer could interpret the effect for themselves within their own field of vision, and come more closely into the experience of the painter.

It was an attempt by these artists to paint with light, and also to go beyond boundaries. They tried to break away from the convention of drawing the image as a separate thing, with an outline against another image or background, also defined by an outline. Instead, they painted object and shadows and background as equally important, moving and flowing into each other. They looked at the known world in a new and visionary way. Yet when they presented these works to the public, people were affronted and shocked. Seeing is such a habit: we see what we expect to see and feel afraid to look beyond the conventionally sanctioned reality of the material world as we 'know' it. We know what we expect, and panic if what we see deviates from the norm of accepted reality.

It is a collective agreement that the table is a solid object. If it is suddenly seen from the reality of a higher dimension, with eyes that are developing greater sensitivity because of the expansion and development of vision, it may be perceived as composed of particles of light/energy dancing to its own tune, giving off its own note. It will be singing a different song to the leaf on the tree, or the stone on the earth. Everything in its atomic light-dance is singing its own unique song as its energy particles dance.

Awakening human eyes will begin to 'see' these things very soon. These artists have tried to show you the way. They were alerted to the possibilities of joy in vision, but then found that the public reacted with panic and reviled them. People were shocked when their comfortable world was disturbed. But you will all be disturbed, and you cannot be comfortable in the old world any more.

The world as you know it now cannot stay at its present rate of vibration. The atoms and particles of its structure are beginning to dance and sing at a higher, faster rate. The earth is awakening to a new consciousness and is stretching and yawning and coming into an awareness of its own destiny in joy, and renewed beauty. The planet Earth is on course to awaken to the conscious knowledge of her own beauty and her true and rightful place in God's universe. The Goddess is rebirthing herself, and will 'mother' a new race of beings. A new humanity. You are becoming this new humanity.

The race of humankind will need to harmonise itself – its own physical vibrations, in order to exist on this reborn planet. Constant renewal will take the place of death in the old way. But we will have to be prepared to leave behind the old way – the old body – and the mental concepts which keep the old body in place, for this renewal to happen. Many artists have been preparing the way for this by flooding our consciousness with the visions of a new reality – new possibilities. Artists of all descriptions, film makers, poets, writers, dancers, healers who work with energy medicine, homeopaths, spiritual healers. All this has been coming together to prepare us and to prepare the way for the immense changes which are now upon us.

There are still many who are resisting the new vision, and clinging to what they 'know'. They want to hear the old tunes repeated, to own pictures which copy and represent closely the 'known' world as this gives them a safe and comfortable and sentimental feeling. It will be harder for them to make the adjustment, which they will need to make, as the changes come in. The raising of vibrations cannot be halted. It will... it IS happening, and these resistances can only cause greater disharmony in the ones who resist. That in its turn could bring about some unpleasant symptoms and even some diseases. This causes us great sadness.

We wish to see the changes come about with the greatest ease and smoothness for you all. And many of us now are reaching down to help you make those steps upwards which will begin to feel steeper as we come nearer the top of the climb. You are indeed climbing up a mountain and are very near the peak. The last steps for many of you could be difficult, maybe the most difficult you have ever taken, but at this point we will reach down to you. You will not fall, you will not fail, as you reach out to grasp our hands held out to you in love.

We have come down to meet you: stepped down our energy levels which is also, in some respects, a difficulty, and let us say a test of mastery for us. But we come with such hope to lift you, and all humanity now, into a state of freedom and joy forever.

Love and Light be with you.

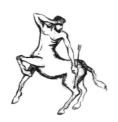

A.Z. SEVENTH COMMENTARY

For some reason I have found the return to this period of my life somewhat more difficult than I had expected. I have always looked back on these days, and envied my younger self for the chance some providence had given us: setting us down amidst the vistas of Queen's Gate and Exhibition Road, with Hyde Park and the Serpentine at one end, and the colleges and museums at the other, and for the wonderful access it gave us to the treasures of our national heritage, and the temples of culture and learning. But I have found myself, instead, unearthing some areas of past experience which have lain in the twilight of consciousness for too long.

Just before contacting A.Z. to ask if he had another comment, I took out a pack of angel cards and drew one. These are tiny cards each with a delightful picture of an angel representing angelic qualities, such as Healing, Trust, Brotherhood, Communication, Adventure, Love. By picking one blind, but intuitively from the pack, the Angelic quality which resonates within you at that moment, will be drawn to you. I drew the Angel of Gratitude, and I spent a moment meditating on that and attuning myself to that Angel's energy, wondering what its message might mean. There *was* much to be grateful for in those years I had just been recalling, but the stress and pain I had experienced in the telling of it, when some of the undealt-with stuff began to emerge from wherever it was I had hidden it, made me wonder just what the Angel was telling me.

You have been looking into and attempting to write about some very difficult areas of your life; areas which have caused blockages in your creative energy – in the expression of that energy. You were under great pressures and constraints at this time in your life. The Angel of Gratitude has appeared to you and that is significant. It could be she will help you to see some of the less obvious aspects of gratitude.

Maybe you felt under constraint to be grateful for what you had been given – all that had been lavished upon you, all those experiences which you have been attempting to describe – and which gave you a sense of indebtedness and obligation. The law of Karma has operated throughout human history via a sense of balance and of justice and the need to repay debts, but we are now coming to a place where we need to clear all vestiges of debris from the past so that we can go forward into the new age fresh and clear. So this lifetime, for many of us, will have been chosen as one where we could accomplish that cleansing process for ourselves, and also for humanity as a whole.

When that aspect of the soul which is to take part in another round of physical existence comes in at birth, it has been preparing carefully for the lessons it will need to learn in the lifetime ahead. This preparation will have been overseen by the Higher Self and undertaken in the company of its spiritual family, those elder brothers and sisters which some of you call guides. The soul understands the need to grow and evolve throughout this learning process, and it sees what debts need to be repaid. This is a complex concept and to simplify it I use the term 'debt', though I don't want to sound negative or judgmental. Don't be daunted by the term 'complexity' either. It should be seen in a most positive light, for the existence of complexity implies that there is unlimited freedom of expression for you to explore and master.

We have talked before of the importance of gaining a sense of balance – balancing acts. One of the great lessons for the soul, as it partners the personality in the body in its earthly life, is to master this area of balance. Repaying debts incurred in former lifetimes is one aspect of balance. Another is to redress the masculine/feminine balance that has been lost when the male has taken too much power and the female has given away too much power.

Both of these aspects you have undertaken in this lifetime. It is very difficult, sometimes, to retain the vision which the soul had at the start of another mission to Earth, when it knew the score, and knew the significance of some of the painful experiences it might find itself in. We get so drawn into earthly experiences and into the personality, its survival strategies and emotions, that we lose sight of our balancing mission. We also lose sight of the support and help we can call upon in the world above.

When we lose, as most of us unfortunately do in these materialistic times, the contact with our spiritual origin, and the knowledge of ourselves as unlimited spiritual beings rather than limited physical beings, the perspective and objectivity about what is happening to us down on Earth gets lost, and we become sucked into seeing events from the perspective of the ego-personality, and react from the ego to the situations we find ourselves in.

116

If we no longer have contact with our Higher Selves and our spiritual family, or the supportive love and power which flows from the Source, then we feel bereft of love and security, and we look to our fellow brothers and sisters on Earth to supply that love. The desire for fame and fortune is also a longing for love and approval. The applause of an audience is as warm sunshine to us and, when an audience or a following praises us for our creations and becomes devoted to us, we feel that warm glow in our hearts.

Of course it is not just the ego that is involved. As I am sure you have observed, the extent of ego-tripping, as I think you call it, varies from person to person. To some extent we all have a joy in being creative, and in creating something of wonder and beauty, and we feel moved by the response of others. We feel moved when we evoke deep feeling or pleasure in others, because we are sharing ourselves with them. Most human beings feel great pleasure when they can give and share something they have created which enhances the life of someone else. It can be as simple as baking a delicious cake, or a salad; it can be that we uplift someone through an act of healing or by singing a song. The joy of creating is magnified in the act of sharing.

But it is the ego which feels anguish when it cannot find the means within itself to create an offering or product which will have the desired effect. It aims to please and cannot find the means, the skill, the talent within itself to create that thing which its patron or client will acclaim. This is the heartbreak of the would-be artist, or for that matter, the lover. 'I am not beautiful enough,' might be the epithet that covers both cases. 'I am not good enough, and the object of my desire, be it client, or lover, rejects me.' This is what we feel and we try harder and harder to please, and in so doing, begin to betray our true self.

I try to make myself 'that which I am not' in order to be approved of and rewarded. And so, sadly, we go further and further away from our true nature, which is spontaneous and joyful, and we become artificial. It is strange, is it not, to see how the word 'artifice' is derived from 'art'? Being artificial and artful are the more negative aspects of creativity. Yes, of course, those practising artifice will often become successful in that and reap rewards, but the connection with the soul grows ever more far apart and the connecting tissue, if I can put it that way, becomes more rigid and unfeeling and the life-blood no longer circulates between the separated halves of the being.

I will now come back to your questioning and wonderings about why you had been given so much; and why, when it seemed you had attained a place in the company of artists of promise and fame, you began to feel such a sense of failure and inadequacy. Why did you feel that you lacked the skills you wished to possess, and were falling short of the standards you desired to reach? I'm afraid it may be that these had been withheld from you in this lifetime for good reasons. Reasons which you once knew.

You were indeed an artist in a previous lifetime. One of much power and skill. A man, arrogant and perhaps somewhat ruthless in pursuit of success. If these very skills and gifts had been granted to you again this time on Earth, you would have become again a successful artist. Not necessarily a ruthless one, for you would have learned something from your previous experience, but becoming a figure of some renown, you wouldn't have been able to put into effect the balancing act which you came here to accomplish. This was not what you were about in the context of this lifetime.

In this life you were granted all the trappings and all the privileges of an artist's life for some time, but you had to break away from it all in order to fulfil another task. You have suffered much pain in all of this, but I have always been by your side, although you did not know it. I have watched you endure what you had to, and have felt 'pain' in a sense while I watched you suffer. Though we don't have the same emotional or bodily sensations as you do in the physical world, I can't find a suitable word to express the 'painful concern' which we, on this side, have for our brothers and sisters on Earth when we see you make mistakes and suffer. You are very dear to us.

The debts that you personally undertook to repay are settled now, and you have a chance to heal the wounds of your life, and enter fully into the role of the Wounded Healer. This is an archetypal role, a sacred calling to service for humanity, in which you join a band of dedicated brothers and sisters who are both in the world of the spirit and also on Earth. This is the task you have undertaken for this lifetime and are fulfilling very well. New knowledge and new horizons are opening up to you which would never have been possible if you had played once again the role of successful artist.

You have for instance, made contact with the Devic Kingdom and with Chiron, the archetype of the Wounded Healer. All this opens up for you now and much more is to come.

I was very grateful for this communication, and after pondering on it for some time, it made a great deal of sense. But I still had the feeling that I had taken it in and understood it in my head, without feeling that anything had changed on the inner level regarding what the ego is craving, while the artist is creating. Both these things seem to be tangled up with one another. So I put this to A.Z. for a further thought.

Yes. This is something very complex, and very much, as you once remarked, like a ball of wool with many threads tangled together. So this is a little job for you to begin to untangle. You may find that one of the threads is that you have this tendency to draw into yourself negative scenarios. Beliefs such as 'I can't', 'I'm not capable', 'I'm not good enough'.

Another part though, is that you needed to experience a breakdown into illness in order to break through into a knowledge of your ability to heal, which then opened up new dimensions for you. You chose to come down at this time, when the great Changes were underway, to be a worker for the Light: you needed to use your creativity in a more integrated way which spanned both the physical and the spiritual world. This step forward in your process towards a 'Master's degree' was to learn, or begin to learn, the art of Spiritual Alchemy: infusing matter with spirit and transmuting the body into light.

My love shines ever with you.

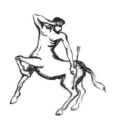

ROAD TO ROME

In spite of increasing doubts about the direction my work would take, I left college filled with a strong current of optimistic, upward surging energy: a momentum which, in my imagination, would lead to a brilliant future living the life of a creative artist, partnered by some handsome and supportive mate. Who that one might be was still undecided, since although it was assumed that Brian and I were more or less wedded to one another, this was not the case. I wasn't at all happy that our relationship was so taken for granted, and felt the need for exploring other possibilities. The thought of settling down was anathema to me, as was the thought of finding a job.

I couldn't envisage my present lifestyle coming to an end, and I wanted only to continue as a carefree venturer. I saw further peaks and capitals ahead, and even as I left the Royal College I entered for more scholarships. I made an application for the Prix de Rome and sent portfolios towards Italian and Greek travelling scholarships. I was shortlisted for the Prix de Rome in sculpture, and given a life-sized set work to complete entitled 'Youth', which was to be exhibited in six months time. Out of ten or so on the shortlist, one would be chosen and awarded two years at the British School in Rome. What possible dream could exceed this prospect?

I had developed a love affair with Italy ever since my first adventure abroad with a girlfriend when I was eighteen. With the magnificent sum of £25 in our pockets, we had hitch-hiked across France hoping to get as far as Rome. We only managed to reach Genoa before the money ran out and we had to turn back, but it was a memorable adventure taking nearly five weeks of the summer vacation. I had met the handsome Roman, Andrea, in some youth hostel in northern Italy where, on a warm, dark evening lying on the grass, with the fragrant pine trees behind us, he had serenaded me with a guitar, while another equally handsome youth had sung a haunting song about a green moon, Verde Luna.

In a pink romantic haze we swapped addresses. Afterwards, when I got back home, the two faces blurred and merged into one and I wasn't sure which of them it was that I was writing back to. It hardly mattered, since it was Italy and the heady prospect of one day meeting up in Rome, that I was falling in love with. Nevertheless a steady correspondence developed, and I allowed an entirely fantastic, idealised romance to build up in my mind. I slept with the letters under my pillow and contrived a fantasy world where this unreal affair could exist. Two years after the first meeting I returned to Italy and met Andrea in the flesh once again. The Eternal City was gradually becoming the goal of my life, since Andrea did not entirely disappoint, and in fact proved to be almost as attractive in reality as he had been in my head.

But the city itself had an even more powerful effect. It was as if I was being drawn there by some inner call. Drawn back to my spiritual home in some inexplicable way. So my bid to gain the Prix de Rome scholarship at the end of my college course took on a desperate quality. Brian had achieved a good degree, and on top of that had been awarded an Abbey Major scholarship which he chose to use travelling and painting for a year in France. The same year that I was working in my studio on 'Youth', the set piece. Brian and I were nevertheless missing each other, and during that time I received a wealth of letters from France imploring me to come and join him. I was torn by a sense of loyalty and deep sisterly feelings for him, yet I knew that I neither loved him nor wanted to marry him.

His letters had become increasingly passionate and I have to say, obsessive and possessive. In that last year he had developed a savage conviction that he could win me by sheer determination, and will me to love him. Just as his sexual behaviour had begun to repulse me by its heavy insistence, so that I reacted to his intimate presence with a physical sensation of suffocation, his ardent letters, even accompanied as they were by beautiful pocket sized semi-abstract paintings of Provence, left me feeling cold and threatened. I was closing down: pulling down the shutters against him in order to defend myself. And I was doing this for one simple reason: I couldn't bear to hurt him by telling him I didn't love him, and that I was allergic to his physical presence.

My inner world was in crisis during this year after I left college, and I came as near as I have ever done in my life to losing my sanity. I was tortured by a fearful sense of shame and guilt brought about by the religious beliefs I still held. Believing on the one hand that if I were to allow another person, other than the first to have broached my virginity, to make love to me, that would amount to the sin of adultery, and the contradictory, but equally devastating realisation, that the God I had believed in as a child was nothing but make-believe. This led to an irreconcilable tension. However illogical it now seems, I was convinced that I was heading for damnation, yet condemned and sent there by a God my rational mind could not and did not believe in.

The Christian upbringing I had been inculcated with emphasised the split between body and spirit. The body was the temple of the spirit, but of itself it was something unworthy and impure. All sensations of pleasure stemming from natural desires were to be denied or controlled in order that the body might become a fit vessel for the spirit to dwell in. I had read Saint Paul and his admonitions, which taught that sexual desires were equated with the fires of lust, and a person dedicated to God must strive to overcome his fallen nature. If they still 'burned', as he put it, then they would have to resort to marriage. But even that prospect held out little attraction for an independent, creative woman. 'As Christ is the head of the church, so man is the head of woman and the wife is subject to her husband and must obey him in all things,' was the blunt misogynist message.

My mind vacillated between belief in this fearful misogynist God and his unacceptable laws, and the equally unacceptable prospect of a desolate wasteland where no God existed and life had little meaning without a spiritual dimension. Every instinct within me told me that I was eternal spirit, yet I was impaled upon horns. I had a choice between a heavenly existence which would have been a personal hell, and the rationalist's, materialistic life which would inevitably end in oblivion.

This agonizing dilemma brought me to the point of breakdown and I fell prey to hallucinations. I began to see devils in every shadow, and random snatches of radio broadcasts started to beam out coded signals at me. Telegrams from hell. Innocuous posters in the street I misread. They became messages personally aimed at me, spelling out the traps set for the unwary sinner. In the pages of the bible itself, I was warned that a slip of the tongue, or a word spoken in jest could precipitate one into a situation where one could commit the unforgivable sin, blaspheme against the Holy Ghost, and find oneself beyond the power of God to forgive, eternally damned. With all this paranoid delusion going on in and around me, it seems a miracle that I was also managing to function in the rational everyday world at the same time. But I took small jobs to make ends meet, and I worked in my studio on my sculptures for the scholarships I was hoping to win. Swinging between normalcy and bouts of mental instability and depression, the year went on.

I shared a studio with a friend, Rose. She was a painter, just graduated from the Royal College like me, who was also working hard on material for similar scholarships in Greece and Italy. One lunchtime we were tucking into our usual steak and kidney pudding in the working men's caff across the road from the studio. I was temporarily back to my normal self and in top form this day. We were deep in salacious gossip and hilarious conversation, and I was telling her the latest joke. Rose had been brought up with ultra strictness in a family of Plymouth Brethren, and I knew she would appreciate this story because it was rather outrageously sexual and anti-religious. I was coming to the point of the story – the punch line.

The Virgin Mary was out shopping with a friend. They stopped by the window of a butcher's shop. In the window was an enormous salami sausage. The biggest either of them had ever seen. 'Oh look!' said Mary, 'It's the Holy Ghost.'

I was in full flow, but realising the import of what I was about to say, I felt the words coming out of my mouth, and saw that I was about to commit blasphemy, but couldn't stop myself. I felt myself metaphorically take a step and place my foot onto ground which immediately gave way, precipitating me down a chute and into the bottomless pit. I felt sick. For days, weeks, I couldn't eat, and soon lost weight and became anorexic. Suddenly there was no point in continuing life. Even less point in ending it. No way forward, no way back. I was a living, breathing impossibility. I felt anger, rage with this God whose stupid laws had brought me to this point.

How was a person to get out of this fix? Slowly, gradually, it began to resolve itself. Damned I might be, but the sun still shone, the birds sang, the bees buzzed, my hair grew. I was still alive and flowers still gave their perfume. I would defy this stupid God and go on living my life, keeping faith with myself. I would be true to *my* truth. I would be sincere, I would honour life all around me. I would do good where I could, or fail where I couldn't, not because Ten Commandments decreed it, or Holy Writ demanded it, but because I was following my innate sense of rightness. I would go on with my work and my plans to get to Rome. So I took a new step forward. It was a strange sensation. I felt fragile, quite insubstantial, but new born.

I plucked up courage one day in Finches bar, our local watering-hole where most of Chelsea's artists congregated, and asked the sculptor whose work I most admired in the world, Elisabeth Frink, to be my sponsor for the Italian Scholarship. Surprisingly, she agreed. She visited me in my work-room, climbing slowly and heavily, as she was in the late stages of pregnancy with her first child, up the stairs to the very top of the building in the Kings Road where Rose and I had our studios. She brought her mother along, a woman I found to be equally extraordinary, equally interesting. Together they went through all my drawings and photographs. With this encouragement and support and the promise of a reference, I set my mind and will on getting to Rome come hell or high water!

From then on I concentrated on finishing my project, *Youth*. The image I had in mind was based on the human figure, but incorporating intuitive elements of my own feeling about the theme. The title I was interpreting *felt* to me like an uncoiling energy. *Spring* perhaps. I began by welding together an inner matrix of iron bars on which I could build up the figure bit by bit, using thick, creamy lumps of plaster mixed with glue size to slow down its setting time, and bulked out by plaster-soaked straw or wood-wool. I felt the figure growing outwards from the matrix energy at the centre. As the work progressed, I followed my inner perception of how my concept would materialise and metamorphosise. Its surface should evoke an aspect of the element of earth. I felt the figure's strength, the masculine strength of *Youth*, as rock, so that he was at once both vulnerable, destructible, flesh and blood and hard, fortress-like, adamantine. The vision that was coming to birth was so complex, so multi-dimensional that I felt I had bitten off more than I could chew. It would need a longer gestation than I had been allowed. Time was ticking away and I had to compromise in order to get it finished. The result was unsatisfactory. Outwardly, it was far from my inner vision, which was still struggling to come to birth. But there was a deadline to meet.

I managed to get the last bits of plaster on just in time to begin colouring the surface with bronzes and greens. The colouring was effective and with that I was pleased, but it was still wet and tacky on the morning set for its delivery. Breathlessly I ran up the road to a local furniture delivery firm and hired a removals van to transport it to the Imperial College gallery, where it was to join the ten or so other exhibitors to be judged and put on public view.

I waited for what seemed an eternity for the results to arrive in the post. I had come second! Seen objectively it was a result not to be sniffed at, but it didn't carry the vital remuneration which allowed the lucky winner to live for two years, with studio provided, at the British School. I was told in confidence later by one of the judges that he had strongly fought my case against the winner, a student from the Slade. They were almost swayed to place me first, but the honour had gone to the Royal College the previous year and they thought it was the turn of the Slade this time. It was a hard blow and it looked as though I had come to the end of the road.

I tried to turn my thoughts to mundane realities. I must find a proper job. But my fervent longing to reach my Everest still burned and would not be quenched. The British School at Rome, high on the Villa Giulia, was the goal of my ambition. Rose had won a painting award and I was pleased at her well deserved luck. She was full of happiness, but disappointed at the same time because I would not now be joining her.

A letter came from Sheffield. I was overwhelmed when I opened it and read its message. 'We're both proud of you and what you have managed to achieve since you left home,' my parents wrote. 'We know how very disappointed you must be not to get selected for the prize and send you this as a token of our love.' It was a cheque for £100. It seemed a staggering amount of money for them to afford. If I could add £50 or so to it by taking a temporary job for a few weeks, I could travel to Rome with Rose after all, and live there until the money ran out.

* * *

The six months that I spent in Rome have to be the climactic experience of my life. Never have I felt more alive, more filled with vital energy, more in tune with my surroundings, than I did in that Mediterranean capital. I stayed for a short time at the British School on the hill above the Villa Giulia, and afterwards shared a room in the Via dei Condotti with Rose. Later Andrea found me a single room on the top floor of one of the shops in the Via Frattina. It had a view looking right down upon the Spanish Steps *and* it was very cheap! The Via Frattina is one of the most prestigious streets in Rome and one would pay a king's ransom for a place there today, but in 1958 I managed to live on L12,000, the equivalent of £7 a week, and pay two of those pounds in rent for a tiny room with a bed, a table and a bowl and jug of water to wash in. I cooked my one good meal a day on the gas ring in my landlady's kitchen, where I learned from her the art of healthy Italian cooking on a shoestring.

Gradually, my inner torment and the paranoia which had dogged me in London, began to abate in the healing warmth of the sun. I was in the very heart of the Holy City, where I had expected to find uprightness and piety, yet all around me was religious and sexual hypocrisy, and political corruption. Somehow that made me feel better. If God was about to damn me to hell for my paltry misdemeanours, then he would have obliterated Rome long ago with a Divine thunderbolt, I thought. The Vatican was rife with scandal. I had witnessed priests creeping out at night through the darkened streets to assignations in brothels. On my first day down at the beach near Fregene the corpse of an attractive woman had been washed up that morning. It was in all the papers the next day, and a bad stench of corruption began to emerge. The press went to town on the story of the 'goings on' in the Vatican. How secret parties, where celebrated models and society women were brought in for the entertainment of the cardinals, had got out of hand. How blackmail and hush-money and finally 'the doing away with evidence so she couldn't talk and give the fun and games away,' had led to this woman inconveniently turning up strangled in the sea. All this was a three day paparazzi wonder, and maybe none of it was true, but the resigned amusement of the local populous who had heard it all before, helped me to shake off the fit of religious self-flagellation I'd arrived with. Above all, I think, it was a discovery I made one day walking down an unfamiliar street. Standing cheek by jowl, joined like Siamese twins, were the Banco di Santo Spirito and the Cinema di Santo Spirito. The incongruous picture it conjured up – the Holy Spirit owning a bank and a cinema – put my little sins finally into perspective.

All in all it was a blessed time, and perhaps the greatest blessing was the fate that had sent Andrea to me. I had gone there with the romantic picture of him still alive inside me. Nothing would have delighted me more than to have ended my time there with a proposal of marriage from him. It would have ensured for me a life in that magnificent city of sunshine and fountains, parks and stupendous ancient architecture. However, the fantasy figure I had fallen in love with began to dissolve quite quickly as I got to know him now on a daily basis, causing me a great deal more painful inner searching and emotional readjustment. But surely it must have been some other-worldly intervention that had provided me, through him, with a complete guide to Rome?

Andrea's studies at University had been long and protracted, as was the custom with the Italians. You studied for a few weeks at a time as and when you could afford it. His subjects were English literature and Roman and Etruscan history. To pay for it, he hired himself out, mainly to Americans, as a guide of Rome. He knew the history of every alleyway and causeway, he was intimate with every tomb and catacomb. There was not a statue, column, nor pillar we did not see. He made it a matter of personal honour to take me into every temple or church, every nook and cranny of his city. We never used public transport, he was as poor as the proverbial church mouse and he walked me to a standstill. When we paused for breath, he would treat me to a couple of lire's worth of salted squash seeds in a screw of paper.

At eighteen, when I had first met him, his tanned skin was set off by a yellow tee shirt and sky blue shorts, but now in the autumn six years later, he embarrassed me by dressing in some terrible zoot suit given to him by one of his American clients in lieu of payment, and looked a fright. He thought he looked the bee's knees. Yet through him I was granted access to a panoramic spread of history and the spirit of the Roman world: deep underground sacred springs, a primitive Neolithic altar, supreme feats of Roman engineering, impressive sculptures, sites of barbaric cruelties juxtaposed with Imperial magnificence, and rising out of Caesar's pagan past, the splendours of Renaissance and Baroque churches.

126

WINGED VISIONS AND A GREEN POPE

The summer season came to an end – the tourists left. As Rose and the others began their first term at the British School, I explored alone, drawing, painting and filling sketch-books with studies from museums and streets. I had an international students card which gave me free access to the inspiring Museo Nazionalle and the Etruscan Museum and all the other places which charged entry, and so I filled my days and my sketch-books. I drew alone among the many ancient ruins of the city, and shared my lunch with the thousands of feral cats, which make their homes there. I made colour studies among the streets of Trastevere, attracting small crowds of onlookers, and spent solitary days amid the ruined ancient Roman cities down by the coast, with the sea wind and the scorpions as company. And I sauntered in silence and dazzling sunlight along the Appian Way.

As I drew and painted, I absorbed. In October, the outdoor markets and shops in the street below my garret room became hung about with furred and feathered creatures. Deer and boar, and birds from the tiniest linnet to quail, were laid out on stalls. I was ambivalent about this. I would linger by the stalls and stroke the feathers of these tiny dead birds. I could never have bought one to eat, yet I had just been invited to a meal at the American School. After drinks we had visited the art studios and met several painters. I was surprised to find that there was a department for film studies too, and we had some stimulating conversations with budding directors, cameramen and musicians. Afterwards, at the meal, we were presented with a plate on which reposed two small winged creatures, seasoned and roasted for our delectation. I was so hungry by then that I thankfully devoured what meat I could find on the carcasses. Which wasn't much.

The next day, as I set out to work with my drawing board under my arm as usual, I passed by several shops, the fronts of which were hung with game animals which had been shot the day before, so that their blood dripped onto the pavement and ran in rivulets across it. Serried ranks of dead birds were laid out for the passer by to inspect and prod, as if they were persimmon or pomegranate. I was drawn by a sense of fascination mixed with pity for the slaughter of these innocents. I lingered, stroked and finally bought one. I took it back to my room and laid it tenderly on the table by the window. What I was going to do with it, I didn't know. Certainly not cook it. I spent some time making a detailed colour study, then a more vigorous impressionistic image. As I became absorbed in the creative process and less aware of my outer self, I began tentatively pulling off the feathers with a reverent curiosity. As my fingers plucked, de-feathering and unclothing the bird, the slow and gradual denudation revealed a little body, which to all intents and purposes was a homunculus. As I came to the part of the body where the wing was joined, I felt my astonishment growing, as, in the details of its anatomy, I could see the same humerus, ulna, radius and even finger bones of the human body underlying the wing structure. I became so excited that I set about making sketches over the next few days for a large sculpture based on my discovery. A winged man. However, because I didn't have access to a studio or the necessary materials, I would have to wait until I got back to London to start it. I can still feel the eerie sensation when, on the following Sunday morning, I bought an airmail copy of the Observer from a paper seller at the foot of the Spanish steps. I opened it at the arts pages and saw a photograph from Frink's latest London exhibition. A Winged Man! Not only that, but I later discovered that Michael Ayrton, another well known sculptor, had also been working on a series of figures based on the Icarus/Daedalus theme, at the same time.

* * *

Towards the end of October I had scrawled in my diary in halting Italian, 'Oggi era un nuova Papa'. Two weeks earlier, Andrea and I had stood on the city walls overlooking the Vatican and watched the smoke signals issuing from the chimney of the room where the cardinals were ensconced. They had been voting in the election for the new Pope, and at the end of each day that no decisive vote was reached, they would burn, in traditional manner, their voting papers. The resultant black smoke signalled their inconclusive debate for that day. Then came the white smoke and Angelo Giuseppe Roncalli, Pope John 21st was ushered in, and a new Papal era commenced. The deceased Pope Pious 12th, whose reign, according to many, had been marked by equivocation and a somewhat questionable courage throughout the wartime alliance with Nazi Germany, died on 9th October 1958. He was to be laid in state in an open coffin, and the plan was that the crowds of the faithful would file past the coffin, mourning and paying homage. The body was to be embalmed so that this spectacle could continue for as long as the grieving crowds wished to see him. The embalming process was taking place during the days that the voting was in session, but news began to leak out that something had gone wrong. The viewing was delayed. It was at first rumoured, then the rumours turned to certain public knowledge, that the corpse had turned green! New arrangements had to be hastily put in place and the usual Italian face-saving strategies staged. Maybe the Holy Ghost did have a sense of humour after all!

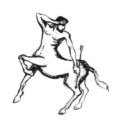

A.Z. EIGHTH COMMENTARY

It is good to go into this part of your life, because so much has happened that was disturbing and heart-rending. I mean that literally. The heart, that is the spiritual or subtle substance of the heart, and in particular the energy centre which we call the Heart Chakra, was torn and damaged at that period. It suffered many blows and tremors and was shutting down. I can 'hear' it now; it is still holding on to those wounds, and you are having difficulty hearing what I am saying to you now, because you don't want to hear it, and that is affecting our lines of communication.

This was true. I was squirming and hearing him indistinctly. It took another year before I could open up enough to write about some of the more painful areas in my life from that period.

The heart feels as if it is in peril and in danger of its very life. It closes shut, but it must open out again to life. It wants you to mend it. It is asking you to heal it, and here is how:

Gradually let it relax and open up. Let my love creep in like sunshine on a spring day. I am the healing light. I want to come in like a bird into her nest; to come to her little ones to nestle them and feed them. Let me into your heart. I long to come into your heart and bring the healing of Love. I have longed to be with you since your life's journey began; hearts entwined. I am your Beloved.

I know what you anticipate – that you are remembering past episodes that took place while in Rome, which shocked and shattered you. You attempted to absorb them and understand and forgive, but you were in such confusion that your feelings were flung into turmoil, and this caused scar after scar to be formed, and there was not opportunity for the heart to be healed. Then, after the damage was done and you closed your heart down, you allowed it to open once more, and gave yourself in love again soon after you returned home. That love was once again betrayed, and the heart was wounded even deeper than before.

As you recount this period, you remember it as a time of Youth and

Flowering and much healing being accomplished, and so it was. But it was also a time of inexperience and callowness, when wisdom was absent. A new set of circumstances was being created and set in motion, which would bring even deeper woundings to your heart. All this has made you unable to trust love again. For you, it became not a healing but a threat and a danger. Yet you longed still, as do we all, for the warmth of love. When you seek love, you are asking for love to exist in you and for you. You are making a declaration of the importance and the existence of love. You recognise its nourishing power and its value.

When we open our hearts to love, it flows in. We see the 'belovedness' of the other, and yet the 'other' fails. He fails because he is human and you are human. Love does not fail. The love that you open to is Unconditional Love. It is the human being who makes it conditional. It is he or she that determines, controls, demands, cheats, exploits and all the rest. You know your need of love, but your friend demands conditions; withholds his love in order to make you do or be something for his ego's sake, and not for your own well-being. But the love of which I speak flows eternally from the Source, it is never withheld from you. The love which flows to you through me is that Unconditional Love. All you have to do is let it in; I am simply part of that love, as you are.

But remember, love cannot fully enter until the hard scar tissue that is protecting/defending your heart gives way. Just let it drop off like dead scales and feel the energy which is flowing in right now as we speak. It is vital, nourishing, life energy that demands nothing in return. You have to become young again, and in order for that to happen, your heart must become flexible and innocent once more. But it will be an innocence that is wiser now. It has learned through its pain and the trauma of betrayal.

The wise heart is young and free. It heals itself so it can be an instrument of healing for others. It has been tempered, now, in the fires of passion and betrayal. The wounded heart can truly sing, for it sings a new note. A clearer, stronger note than when it was untried and untested. The heart is like a bell; its metal has been forged in holy fire. The fire of suffering and grief. Its shattered pieces are come together now and will form a new design.

There was once a beautiful mediaeval stained glass window in a cathedral. In one of those 'holy' wars, vandals and ignorant men smashed it to pieces. The people who had loved it so much gathered the pieces together and commissioned a great artist to put it together again. It was impossible to reconstruct it as before, so he was inspired to create a circular design, a Rose Window, and it became a glorious abstract mosaic of translucent colour. You know how the rose symbolises the heart and is also a symbol for both spiritual and earthly love.

The heart is a bell resounding with pure, delightful sound;
It is a wheel of translucent multicoloured light;
It is a tender, fragrant flower breathing out perfume,
And a nest sheltering little birds.
It is God's chamber of Light and Joy;
In it are all things made whole again.
It is a crucible of Holy Flame and Holy Love;
It is a wise and flexible vessel of great power.

Oh! My little bird, how I wish I could have protected you.
But you would never have grown in beauty, if I had.

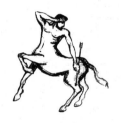

FIVE

THE SICK ROSE

O Rose, thou art sick!
The invisible worm
That flies in the night,
In the howling storm,

Has found out thy bed
Of crimson joy,
And his dark secret love
Does thy life destroy.

William Blake 1757-1827

ENTANGLEMENTS

I had returned to my old shared flat in Chelsea after six wonderful months away in Italy, leaving behind me, even in December, a world of blue skies and golden sunshine. Now I was back in frozen, dismal London, just three days short of Christmas. Before I left Rome, Andrea and I had gone to the Trevi Fountain together and thrown in coins. We'd planned to marry as soon as he could manage to pluck up his courage and leave Mamma. He would join me in London for a while and try to integrate himself with the London scene that had become so important to me. I wanted him to meet my friends and get to know the very different and rather unconventional way of life that I had begun to carve out for myself. A world where, I had pointedly told him, a generation of young artists and other creative thinkers were living lives independent of parent or priest, thinking their own thoughts, and forging a more liberal morality.

In the last five years I had visited Rome three times, but I had never bothered with the tourist ritual of throwing coins in the Fountain to ensure return. But this was a more significant occasion, a sort of commitment, or a plighting of troth, as we had already sought the necessary permission from the authorities for a marriage between a Protestant and a Catholic. I threw in my coin, promising Andrea I would return. I left Rome that day full of anxieties about our frail relationship and the gravest doubts as to whether I was doing the right thing. It was December 1958 – I have never returned.

The twenty-four hour train journey to Paris was a watershed. With each mile Andrea's image grew fainter and my memories of London grew stronger. My thoughts returned to the day I left London. My friend Mahendra had waved me goodbye at Victoria Station. During the time I had last been in London, working on my Prix de Rome piece and the other scholarships, and Brian was away in France, I had met up with a lively contingent of Sinhalese students and artists. The painter, Ivan Perries became one of my greatest friends. He was already an established artist and had represented Ceylon, his country, at the Bienalle in Venice.

They were an extremely talented and sophisticated lot, and far more compatible in their humour and unconventional approach to life than any of the people I'd met in Italy. Mahen was one of the liveliest of them, and a very attractive member of that group, and I had begun to develop a close friendship with him just before I set off for Rome.

The Italian adventure had, without doubt, been an incredibly enriching experience and one I would never regret. Yet I was beginning to realize, more strongly with each mile that passed, how much I had tried to turn myself inside out in the last six months in order to fit in with Roman society. Misgivings flooded in. The contradictions I'd juggled with, as I struggled to be tolerant about the enormous differences I encountered in the lifestyles there. The revelations I had gradually uncovered about the political and religious corruption, and their double standards in sexual matters. Andrea had told me for instance that he had gone regularly to confession and had to admit his guilt about masturbating. The priest had been stern and condemnatory. Self-abuse was a grave sin and forbidden by God, he said, and rather than have this on your conscience causing unbearable sorrow to Him, it would be better to sleep with a girl of the lower classes. 'Your mother has a servant, perhaps? Lie with her. Or do what I do, and visit one of the brothels in town which are vetted by our doctors. They have healthy women there, and we teach them to fill their vaginas with water so that sperm will be washed out and not be likely to cause pregnancy. Do this my son, but on no account lie with a girl of good family and breach her virginity before marriage. Above all, do not abuse yourself.'

I tried to be more accepting about these cultural differences, but it had cost me too much in self esteem and respect. As each mile of the journey took me further from Rome and nearer to London, all this hit me with the shock of clarity. The train track, the insistent rhythm of the metallic wheels speeding northwards, was reconnecting me with my familiar self once again. Then as I stepped onto the platform at Victoria a few days later, struggling with my heavy suitcase, Mahen, with total unexpectedness, stepped out of the crowd and was at my side.

We hadn't corresponded all the time I was away. When he'd waved me goodbye at that same station, I assumed that would be the end of our growing attachment, and that he would resume his life and his other relationships. It was a sad and painful moment, but there it was! I was off on an adventure of my own and I managed to put him out of my mind. But now he was here, running towards me. 'I've missed you every day, every moment you have been away. Couldn't wait for you to come back.' he said. And incredulously, I felt my heart leap at his words. The flame was rekindled instantly.

He was then about twenty four, the same age as myself, and had been studying law at Gray's Inn for some years. He had come here from Sri

Lanka, or Ceylon as it was then, when he was quite young. Although precocious in his abilities, and one of the youngest students ever to come from abroad and to be accepted at Gray's Inn, he was not cut out to be a lawyer. Although he had been brilliant as a young scholar, now on the eve of every exam he would go down with a fever and be incapable of sitting it. It wasn't that he lacked the capacity to pass the exams, it was simply that he feared having to follow in his father's footsteps, which led into the legal profession. He was by temperament an artist, but sadly he didn't have the necessary talent for this calling, so he lived the artist's life and funked the law exams. Unable to create himself, he encouraged, supported and inspired others and myself in particular. His knowledge and taste was highly developed and sophisticated. His interests were wide and we found we had a great deal in common.

One of my heroes in those days was Father Trevor Huddleston, who was at that time working in the townships with black South Africans. Once, I had seen his photograph in a paper, and had been so attracted to his characterful appearance that I had used him as a model for one of my sculptures. Then a year or two later, whilst I'd been at the British School, I had discovered his book *Nought for Your Comfort* in the library. After reading it, I became more deeply involved than ever in the Anti-apartheid Movement, which was one of the causes close to Mahen's heart, and one which he tirelessly worked for. We were also enormously concerned by the threat of The Bomb, which overshadowed everyone's lives with fear. Mahen was an energetic organiser, and was involved with the Aldermaston marches. We marched side by side in the second march, which went from Aldermaston to Trafalgar Square. It was a gesture of commitment which we passionately (but naively, as it turned out) felt would move the Powers That Be to disarm and live together in peace.

We found that we shared many more passions and concerns. There were magazines publishing new poets, there were the new and influential plays of the late fifties: Joan Littlewood at the Theatre Royal, Stratford East, and the *Angry Young Men* in Sloane Square, not to mention Ionesco and Beckett. There was the National Film Theatre and the South Bank, there were jazz clubs and music at the Festival Hall. Mahen had a young cousin, Rohan de Saram, the cellist. Rohan had been one of that rare group of beings, an infant prodigy, and by one of those uncanny coincidences, he had been born, almost by accident, in Sheffield. His parents happened to be staying with Dr. Perera, his uncle, who had a long established general practice there. As a child of three or four, and back by now at his parents' home in Ceylon, he had been summoned to play for Mary, the old Queen Mother, when she was on a visit to that country. Later he was taken on by the great cellist, Pablo Cassals, as a pupil. We once went to one of Rohan's concerts at the Queen Elizabeth Hall, and found ourselves, with some surprise, sitting in the row just behind the High Commissioner for Ceylon and his guest, the young Prince Charles!

Then there was the exciting world of Soho pubs and clubs where the artists, poets and writers would meet, and suddenly I was back in the swing of pre-Swinging London; and how I had missed it! We went, Mahen and I, to parties and we flirted; sometimes with one another, sometimes with old friends, sometimes with strangers. But without intending to get into deep or serious feelings, an intense attraction was developing between us. We were invited to the same lively gatherings, where cheap wine would be flowing, jazz music beating off the walls and ceilings, and tight groups of people intensely engrossed in art talk. We would be in the same room trying to be casual and giving the impression that this emotional chemistry between us had no reality. Separated by dozens of closely packed bodies, it nevertheless seemed that the very air had caught fire, connecting us and joining us as if we were standing body to body. From opposite sides of the crowded room, through the dim, party-time light, we felt ourselves lit up by the same invisible, magnetising beam, and conscious of the other's presence to the exclusion of everyone else. We fought against it, flung ourselves into animated conversations and danced with other people, but the magnetism was too strong, it kept on pulling us together and bumping us into each other.

Apart at night we could not sleep; going about our business in the daytime – perhaps setting out to visit a friend across London, or a trip to an art gallery – we would find one another on the same bus, as if some telepathy had alerted us and set us on an inevitably converging path. Neither of us wanted this to happen. Both had enough entanglements with other relationships and other commitments.

Curiously, I had heard nothing of Andrea since we parted on the railway platform in Rome. Secretly I was glad; I didn't know what to say to him. Then one day the postman delivered a heavy envelope which contained a lengthy letter from Andrea's mother. She had gone to the trouble of getting someone to write it for her in English, so I knew it was going to be serious. With so much excitement going on for me in London, and not knowing how I could possibly explain all that had taken place to Andrea, I had been relieved not to have heard anything from him for some time, but his mother's letter brought me up with a start. Andrea, it seemed, had been subject to great anxieties and doubts about coming to London. The thought of leaving his mother and venturing abroad into unknown territory to make his fortune and try to prove himself to me, had caused him to succumb to a nervous breakdown and he was now in a 'House of Restoration' in the countryside being tended by the nuns!

I experienced a gamut of conflicting emotions. I was genuinely concerned for him; I was twisted up with guilt; but most of all I experienced relief, when I understood that what she was really saying was that he wanted an honourable get-out from the promises we had made to each other of marriage.

Shortly afterwards, Mahen and I were sitting in a café in the Fulham Road. We had been lingering over a cup of coffee, aware that people were coming and going, ordering their meals, eating and departing again, while our cup of coffee, like the cruse of oil in the bible, seemed miraculously never to dry up. We were so wrapped up in one another that the energy field surrounding us seemed to belong to a different time from the rest of the world. We hadn't spoken for ages; hardly moved. Gazing into each other's eyes, which had deepened and opened to one another, so that we'd become drawn into a single heart beat, this ecstatic wordless, timeless, passionate moment flowed on. Mahen, playing with a long gold chain, which I wore around my arm, slowly began to untwist it then twist it again, round and round our two wrists. One dark hand, one light hand, symbolically joined in a golden band.

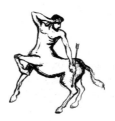

A BIRTH, A DEATH AND A NAMING

A palpable power now joined us, we were two halves of one being, and yet there was something more – perhaps it was Unity itself which we sensed as a third force. All the inhibitions I had felt during my long relationship with Brian had gone. That physical incompatibility, which he had regarded as frigidity on my part, melted away. I was surprised at myself, surprised how responsive I was finding myself to be to physical passion. For it was true, I was experiencing that sensation we call love, and the full return of the same feeling for the first time. For Mahen, too, was a person transformed. All his outward, cynical, defensive cleverness had dropped away and he was revealing a vulnerable, sensitive inner reality.

He told me stories of his childhood in Ceylon. How the British troops had been stationed there and how badly they had behaved, but in comparison with the Japanese their behaviour faded into insignificance. As a small child, he had always loved to go by himself into the jungle and watch the wildlife, and once came upon a group of soldiers firing off their machine guns just for the hell of it, slaughtering everything in sight, in the trees, in the streams, in the bush. Thousands of dead creatures everywhere. He was moved as he told me, and then became ashamed of his emotions. He told me of his love for the elephant. How, in contrast to the image most people had of them as lumbering and clumsy, to him they were the most graceful of all God's creatures. He had tremendous respect for them. I could tell he felt that sharing these insights into himself was dangerous. I had got underneath him, touched him inside his armour, and found a loveable but frightened person there.

I was constantly being surprised by what I was discovering in him and in my own feelings, but I must confess I was astonished when he put his feelings into words, and came out with the declaration that he had this longing to plant a baby-seed inside me; half Mahen, half Esmé, as he put it. Until then, I had never had the slightest desire for a baby, nor any hint of maternal thoughts, but his words sparked something in me which must have been lying dormant. Then there came a moment during our love-making when we both recognised that it had happened. We knew it instantly, but it was Mahen who again put it into words.

'Ah! *That was it*. Did you feel it?' he said. 'There is our baby conceived inside you now.' And so it was.

We had entered a world neither of us had previously known. A state made magical by the awakening of deep passionate feelings. One warm night we lay naked together on the bed. Moonlight falling upon soap boxes stuffed with clothes, two broken chairs and a rickety table, which comprised the scant furnishings of the room, cast a transformational spell over all. The pearly light transformed the atmosphere so that we became detached observers of our bodies. 'Look,' he said, as if it was a sculptural composition we were viewing, and illumined by silver-blue we saw one pale, translucent body entwined with another dark body, almost black on the white sheet. And we felt awed by what we saw. Darkness and Light, the Yin and the Yang symbolically holding one another in an embrace.

For a while this magical, sensual state existed. For days and weeks it remained, but of course it couldn't last. We had swung too far into the extreme of passion and feeling, and the discovery that I was indeed pregnant brought us both back to reality with a bump. Mahen began to realise the practical implications of having a wife and child, and how it would look to 'The Party.' That being the Communist Party and the group of left wing Sinhalese revolutionaries he was involved with. They were all embroiled in some sort of political machinations dedicated to the violent overthrow of the ruling élite in Ceylon. I never took them too seriously; but for them this business was deadly serious.

To Mahen himself it represented a Brotherhood to which he had given his total allegiance. In what was to my mind a rather twisted view, he described it as if it were a kind of monastic order to which he had made vows of poverty and obedience, and if not *chastity*, well – he had forsworn marriage – or so he said. When finally he returned to Ceylon, he would dedicate himself to living on a minimal allowance, and one meal a day. At that time, the Prime Minister was Solomon Bandaranaike, and Mahen detested the wealthy, ruling élite who were in power in Ceylon. The fact that his own family were part of that élite, since his mother's cousin was married to the Prime Minister, might have been one of the factors in his identifying himself with the underclasses. There was certainly an idealism which made him want to renounce the privileged position he had been born into. There was some irony, too, in that this second cousin of his, Mrs Sirimavo Bandaranaike was soon to become the world's first woman Prime Minister.

The down-to-earth reality of pregnancy soon doused the bright flames of his love and passion. Whether it was the 'Brotherhood' which exerted its disciplines, or that he panicked himself at the thought of parental responsibility, I don't know, but he began to close up. He donned that rakish, quick-witted, tough persona that he exhibited to his political friends, and took to going out every night, leaving me alone. He became the party-going sophisticate of the art world once again. The sensitive person he had revealed to me in secret, and which I had fallen in love with, retired behind a legalistic mind. Had that sweetness, that nectar of the heart, threatened to drown him so that the last traces of feeling had to be banished? Did he sense love as a trap? Something to be avoided and overcome? It seemed to me tragically that love was still there, but he had deliberately set about killing it off.

* * *

It was March and my twenty-sixth birthday. Brian had come down from Leicester, where he was now teaching at the College of Art, to spend the day with me. In two weeks time I was expecting the birth of the baby, and I was very slow and heavy. Brian and I saw quite a lot of each other still, and he and Mahen had developed an uneasy friendship in which there was a lot of mutual respect, but also a wariness regarding their relationship to me. On the surface we were all very civilised, very tolerant and denying of jealousy, while underneath there was a turmoil of conflicting emotions.

Mahen and I were still living together in the orange-box, tea-chest furnished flat in my friend's house at the Angel, Islington. There was one cold tap for all our washing. It was in the attic and it was impossible to stand up straight to use the sink because it was under the angle of the roof. But the rent was minimal: £2.00 per week as a concession for looking after my friend's small child on the days she taught at yet another Art School. These last weeks before the baby was due were becoming difficult and tiring, as I was constantly climbing the several flights of stairs with heavy shopping or five gallon cans of paraffin for our stove. The arrangement to look after the little boy was also causing stress.

Mahen was out at one of his meetings, as he was most of the time, and had hardly acknowledged that it was my birthday. But Brian and I spent a warm, happy day together. He celebrated my birthday by cooking us a meal strongly influenced by culinary skills he had learned while he was in France. Then he had to go, and I spent the late afternoon and the evening seeing to the needs of the little boy downstairs. Exhaustion overtook me, and I longed for little Jay's bedtime so that I could go back to my attic flat and put my legs up. I heard Mahen come in but he didn't look in on me, and I was too tired to call him. At long last Jay was ready to go to bed. I dressed him in his nightclothes and lifted him up with one last effort over the high rails of his cot and put him into bed. I had to lift him high because the mechanism on the cot rails was jammed. As I lifted him up with my arms outstretched, I felt something go snap inside.

I got to the foot of the staircase somehow, but I had no strength left to climb up, and helplessly half sat, half lay in the hallway for quite some time. At long last I managed to attract Mahen's attention and he found me soaked in thick salty water. The waters had broken. After lazily keeping well out of the way until then, avoiding having to find out how I had been coping with my day or offering me help, he now moved into action, phoned the hospital, bundled me into the van, and drove at speed to the Royal Free Hospital. Labour had begun. It was traumatic and painful, but fairly short, and around 4 a.m. that morning a tiny girl, perfect as a china doll, uttered her first cry.

I awoke a few hours later, still in the delivery room, feeling spent and groggy. A brisk and cheery nurse appeared and ordered me to sit up. I weakly told her I couldn't sit up. 'Nonsense,' she said, as is the way of cheery nurses, and she took my arms and pulled me up into a sitting position. I felt the room fading and fell back again in a faint. Soon there was a crowd of medics rushing hither and thither. I had haemorrhaged and lost a lot of blood in the three or four hours since the birth, which no one had noticed.

I was conscious of a lot of pain, and things were getting worse. They were rushing about and soon there was a battery of equipment surrounding me, but I was drifting in and out of consciousness. Consultants were called, matrons summoned. The day wore on and I grew weaker, and my breathing began to falter. I struggled for breath and my lungs started to make strange rumbling and rattling sounds. The blood pressure equipment, with which they tested me every fifteen minutes, showed an alarming drop. My confidence wasn't boosted, either, when they finally let Mahen in to see me, but outfitted in a long white gown and mask. All I could see of him were a pair of dark circled eyes beneath a drawn, anxious forehead, and hands clutching an inappropriate box of chocolates.

As the night passed I was monitored by a relay of junior women doctors who came in dressing gowns and curlers straight from their beds. This relay continued throughout the morning, and at one point the grey-haired midwife who had been present at the birth was taking her turn. She was holding my wrist and keeping her fingers in contact with the faint beat of my pulse. I heard her say to herself, 'It's very faint. I can hardly feel it.' I had been in intense pain, but I was feeling drowsy and welcomed the feeling of drifting off into a reassuring sleep. But the drifting was not turning out to be quite so reassuring. I was floating up-wards into darkness, and it felt as if I was beginning to be sucked or drawn into a long, dark passageway. Then I was being pulled at in-creasing speed along a tunnel, and I thought of Alice in Wonderland and her descent down the rabbit-hole. But I wasn't going downwards; this was a horizontal movement. It grew ever darker and I began to feel afraid.

All my worst fears suddenly surfaced. All the things I thought I had put behind me. The terror of damnation and eternal punishment, which had provoked the episode of near insanity in that year before I went to Rome. The equal fear of oblivion and the finality of death, if, after all, there was no truth in the belief I still clung to of spiritual survival: a be-lief in the soul. I thought I had managed to come to some resolution – equilibrium; some understanding of the crisis of belief which had flung me into that nightmare breakdown some years ago. But as I was drawn and swirled along this dark corridor the blackness grew more intense. And the terror grew more acute also, until I knew I would have to face that fear. 'This is it, then,' I said to myself. 'This is death. Now I shall know if I am to be damned by this irrational God who can't forgive a joke, or if I am to end in oblivion. Whichever it is, or if it is something else altogether, I will face it now.'

I confronted the terror and entered the ultimate blackness. Almost im-perceptibly at first, it seemed less intense. Now I was *sure* it was less dark. I travelled on and sensed a tiny light. 'It's the light at the end of the tunnel,' I said, aware of the cliché. I was also aware that the light was getting nearer and more distinct, and that my fear was receding as it came closer. Soon I was swirling in an intense white radiance, almost blinded, losing consciousness as I drifted in the light. Gradually my awareness returned and I found myself high above the surface of the Earth. Looking down, I could make out a coastline, some unrecognisable country was below me. I wasn't concerned, nor was I afraid of being at this great height. I found that I was now high over the sea suspended in the blue air and warmed by the sunshine, and completely detached from thought or emotion. Then something stirred and I began remembering where I had come from, and with that, strong images from my life came flooding back along with their emotional context. I was thrown into scenes from my past and the accompanying sensations were acute. Stronger even than when the actual events had taken place on Earth. Like being on some giant dipper at the fairground, I was pitching in and out of a series of life events. Each time I dipped into one of these scenes, I reconnected with possessions that had a special significance. I re-possessed objects from childhood, my collections of coins, shells, pressed wild flowers, dolls and books, feeling the impact of their emotional flavour almost as a taste. But then, as I exited from the scene with the upward momentum of the process, I found myself, as I rose higher and higher, letting go of these things that meant so much to me. The moment the impulse came to drop them I experienced a great sense of loss, almost physical, like a painful wrench. But as the momentum lifted me, the letting go became easier and I noticed that, as the weight of these earthly possessions dropped away, my ascent became freer and more joyful.

The process continued, and each time I swung down again, it was into a different area. The possessions became progressively more recent and more adult until it was no longer material things but situations, life-events which I was required to re-enter. Areas of emotional conflict where pain had predominated. I viewed myself again engaged in passionate arguments about politics; reliving scenes where I had been hurt by feelings of jealousy or betrayal; trying to hold on to Mahen in spite of knowing the relationship could never be harmonious and fulfilling. But also there were areas of fleeting happiness, wonderful moments from the past which I desperately wanted to cling on to. I re-experienced them all with great intensity and then was shot out of them again, rising up and away. As I did so I began to view these episodes in a more objective way, letting them go with a sense of relief. Then intimate moments of relationships were re-experienced; deepest friendships and loves. I felt quite blessed to know them once again, and curiously at peace when I eventually let them go.

This sense of peace and trust enveloped me as I rose higher and higher. I was drifting once again in the lovely, ethereal light, feeling secure, yet glad to have experienced this release from all that bound me to Earth. No more pain, and conscious of nothing but freedom, light and movement. This sense of movement grew stronger, and I began to feel once again that I was being drawn into a vortex and swirled along through a spinning funnel of light. Then I heard faint voices. Strong, beautiful voices, in the distance at first, but gradually, as I was drawn nearer, I could hear that they were calling to me; encouraging me on. I had forgotten now the extraordinary scenes which had just taken place. The usual memory which orients us through time sequences didn't seem to exist. I was now back again in the tunnel in which I had encountered the blackness and the terror, but that was all behind me. My consciousness now surfaced at the point where I had registered the light in the distance and the feeling that I was rushing towards it. Once again I was enveloped in that swirling sea of white light, seeing nothing, helpless, yet curiously no longer afraid. I could hear voices though, and was beginning to catch what they were saying. They were calling my name. Calling to me and saying, 'We're holding out our hands. Let us help you through. Let us help you. We have been waiting for you.'

I held out my arms and they drew me forward. It was as though I myself was being born as I was eased out into a shimmering landscape. All of a sudden I found myself in a field of silvery white grasses moving like the waves of the sea in a gentle, warm, refreshing wind. Then I saw the field was full of daisy-like flowers, silver-white also, and huge, soft and delicate. Everything was luminous, not from a source of light, but everything emitting its own light. Above all, I was light; light as a feather, free and joyous. I had never before felt so happy and I wanted to run all over and through the field exploring this new energy and lightness. I discovered I could fly! I could trail my feet in the pollen of the shimmering white petals and the flowering, flowing grasses. I never wanted to be anywhere else. This was not a dream. I knew, in a way which is impossible to communicate, that this was more *real* than the reality of the body. I was in a new body, or rather I had discarded the old body and had taken possession of my real body.

The delight of this new, strong, and immensely light body was just beginning to dawn on my mind. My conscious awareness was beginning to catch up with the serendipity of finding myself transformed, when I heard a voice and knew that it was not issuing from the plane I was in at that moment. The voices which had called me and helped to birth me into this new world had receded, as if to stand back whilst I got my bearings. I felt their presence near at hand, and even sensed their outstretched arms ready to catch me if I stumbled, but this voice I was hearing now was far, far away, yet it had a familiar ring. I didn't want to have to take notice of it. I strained my new ears and it made me ache in my heart when I realised the significance of those words. It was a woman's voice and she was saying, 'It is very faint.' Then a pause, and, 'Oh my God! It's stopped altogether now.' And I knew it was the grey-haired midwife holding my wrist and feeling my pulse. 'Oh my God,' she said in anguish, 'she's gone now.'

As the words sunk in it struck me for the first time, and with a sense of dismay, that I had completely left that world behind. Left it with joy and relief, and was about to enter an adventure in a new land of exciting freshness and beauty, and creative freedom: I'd just begun to be aware of exciting possibilities opening out ahead of me, possibilities I'd never even dreamed of. But the voice pulled me up, and in a way 'brought me back to my senses', jolting my memory of what had just taken place on Earth in the old world.

A new life. A little baby had just been born in that world down there, was no one to look after it but me. I couldn't leave it to its ,ents or to Mahen's sister. Worst of all, I couldn't leave it to be ֹ t up in a Home. *I must get back.*

Gripped now by this overwhelming urgency, I struggled to detach myself from this new world, just as I had a short while ago from the Earth. This was harder though, and now I had to make a great effort to pull myself back. I let the voice of the midwife guide me, and homed in on her, remembering her as I had last seen her sitting beside my bed. She was still holding my wrist as though I had been away only a few moments! I let this image guide me, and felt myself coming down until I reached what I can only describe as the pain barrier. There was a sense of re-entry into a heaviness and density, and as I came further down I saw my body beneath me. I sensed the pain surrounding that body. I felt it at first as a threshold around the body, so I could feel the pain yet was not *in it.* Though reluctant to enter it again, the pull of the body's energy-field was like a magnet, too strong to resist. I was returning rapidly, but knew I had chosen of my own free will to return to life's pain and responsibilities once again.

My lungs seemed hardly to be functioning. Breathing with the greatest difficulty, I made an effort. I opened my eyes, looked into the face of the midwife and murmured, 'It's all right. I have come back.' She gazed at me, her eyes widening with astonishment and then filling with tears. I found myself breaking into waves of the deepest sobs; total, uninhibited sobbing. I cried out my heart until my lungs faltered, whereupon she reached over, threw her arms around me and sobbed with me.

* * *

This going in and out of time and in and out of different worlds wasn't quite finished with yet. They kept me in the labour ward for another two days after the birth, as I wasn't well enough to be moved, and around me they set up a makeshift intensive care unit. The relay of student doctors continued around the clock, and there was another episode when I relapsed and my lungs collapsed. Again I was surrounded by a battery of breathing apparatus, blood transfusions and other drips and tubes, and I drifted out of consciousness once more. I floated upwards: I seemed to be making a habit of it. This time however, I simply stayed up by the ceiling. (I must make it very clear that at this point in my life I had never heard of 'out of body experiences', nor read anything of that phenomena which is widely reported nowadays.) Up by the ceiling, I gazed down upon myself. It didn't seem strange to be in this position. But I was aware of panic going on. The 'me' down there was going through agonies of pain and anguish, as she realised she was slipping away from her body once again. The nurses and midwives, and junior doctors clustered around the bed, were also in panic. I could hear them shouting at one another, and all making suggestions, which were being contradicted by other opinions. Until at last someone yelled, 'for heavens sake, send for Mr Sheldrake.' He being the great consultant in charge. 'He's on his rounds somewhere down the corridor,' I heard one of them say.

I watched from my exalted position and saw that the great man was indeed coming. I swooped down a little and came nearer to my body, and as I did, I felt myself becoming involved in the sensations of pain and panic again. So I drifted back to the ceiling. Here all was calm and clarity. I listened to the huddle which had gathered by the bed again, this time joined by Mr S and observed their discussion with complete medical knowledge and understanding of all the terms they were using. When they pronounced on the exact dosage of a particular drug, and the administration of morphine or whatever, I knew they had got it right, and that I would survive. I could leave the scene as I knew their patient was in good hands and under the correct treatment. It was as though I had presided over my own case conference. All would be well.

* * *

I was moved to the recovery ward two days later. On her rounds the grey-haired midwife, she who had thrown her arms around me and wept, she who had held my faltering pulse as it faded away to nothing and opened her eyes with astonishment when I announced my re-entry, came in to see me. 'How are we today?' she said. 'Good! Good! You're looking much better. Keep it up.' And with that she swept out again. She didn't look me in the eyes, and there was no trace whatsoever of what had taken place between us. I often wonder how she has explained all of this to herself.

* * *

It was three weeks before they allowed me to leave hospital, during which time Mahen visited me every day, bringing books, relating humorous incidents, keeping me in touch with outside events. One day he came in shaken, to report that a massacre had taken place at Sharpeville when South African police had fired into an unarmed crowd of black men, women and children. But there were lighter moments too, as quite unconsciously, but in a somewhat fairytale fashion, we arrived at a name for our child. On *three* consecutive evenings he brought *three* names for me to consider. European ones came first: Francesca, Julia, Belinda, then Gabrielle, Andrea and Chantelle. I liked these but couldn't decide. The third evening he came with three Sinhalese names, Siriani, Sandhya and Dhevi. I asked what they meant. Siriani was his youngest sister's name and meant 'sugar'. I wasn't so keen when I heard that. Dhevi, with the Sinhalese spelling, meant 'princess' or 'goddess', and Sandhya, he said, meant 'Twilight'. Straight away I loved that and became enthusiastic, even more so when he went on to tell me that there was a Sandhya tree whose flowers opened just as the sun was setting, and gave out a wonderful perfume. Also there is a bird with the same name that begins to sing just as it grows dark and the sun's light fades. 'They call it the Night Bird,' he said wickedly, 'and I dare say any daughter of mine will be a little night bird.'

In spite of his dubious humour, it was decided upon. Eighteen months later I went into Islington reference library to see if I could find out more about the name, and was allowed to take home a Sanskrit dictionary. It was about eighteen inches high and weighed a ton. I searched through it at leisure, and had some difficulty finding the name at first because of the unfamiliar language and alphabet. But when I did find it I felt a tingling all down my back as I uncovered its full meaning.

SANDHYA (the n is pronounced very soft so as to be almost an m.)
Holding together. The junction of day and night. Morning or evening twilight. Dawn.
Goddess of the three divisions of the day; morning, noon, evening.
A meditation enacted at the three points of day; morning, noon, evening.
Sandhya was the daughter of Brahma and consort of Siva, the Sun.
Uniting – Healing – Growing together – Re-uniting – Peace – Friendship.
The point at which union takes place.
The space between heaven and earth:– The horizon.
Produced by coalescence.
Situated at the point of contact.

How had we come to alight on this name for the child of our union? I am sure that Mahen had not known these further dimensions to the name, or how it so significantly expressed the coming together of the Dark and the Light, the East and the West, and the merging of the two cultures.

A.Z. NINTH COMMENTARY

Let us look now at this phase of your life and link it with lives you have lived in other times and other places. I want to regard it in the context of a greater life path; the Soul's journey.

You have linked into Rome and its wider history with the help of your friend Andrea. He enabled you to 'tune in' to the many levels and layers of 'the story that is Rome'. You delved with him into some of its deeper aspects, both in the archaeological sense of going down into progressively deeper layers of its civilisation, and also in the sense of the more dark and negative aspects of its present social and religious orders. This was a necessary undertaking for you.

It was necessary to link with that part of the great civilisation from its foundations upwards. You went deep into its caves and its history. The walls and pillars of that great city hold within them, in their cellular structure, the reverberations of all that has taken place there through the ages. And now the cells of your body have had those vibrations transmitted to them so that they hum with that vibration. Your body has hummed out this tune into the places and the environments into which you have gone since.

It has gone through you, as it were, and like an instrument or sounding board the notes have been amplified, strengthened and transmuted. You have been an instrument, that is, instrumental in making a sound that will help to change the world. Wherever we walk we give out a sound just as we give out a light – contributing to a light network which is strengthening and building the future. It is also a sound network, or a web of sound wave patterns that harmonise with the Universal music making. The music of the spheres.

And so, after that encounter with Rome we come home again to England and pick up where we left off in our relationship with Mahen, the dark partner from the Asian continent. Heaven's above! How fast you moved. What great work you undertook. You didn't know that, did you? You just went gaily on and didn't feel a thing. Unaware how the spiritual choirs were singing as you moved from one sphere to another across

Europe and into Asia with the speed of a twenty-four hour train journey. Carrying all that stuff. All that baggage to transmute.

You didn't know what weights you had lifted. What you had picked up and what you had to shed. You carried one load of baggage back home with you and soon you were reconnecting with Mahen, which put you in touch with another series of lifetimes which you had spent in the Indian subcontinent. A reconnection with more past lives and more cultural baggage.

You felt yourself very drawn to marriage with Mahen because within yourself you had a sense of mission to bring together the two great world cultures: the Western, logical, scientific, male culture, and the Eastern, intuitive, spiritual, sensual, feminine culture, and out of this marriage there would be a Child of this Union.

When two great urges representing polar opposites or dualities come together the Child of this marriage is a Wondrous being – Unity is its name. Unity and Wisdom, Peace and Friendship, is the fruit of the coming together.

Humanity has within itself this split. It has the power of choice and can make decisions and thus experience the one side or the other in depth. Experiencing Maleness or Femaleness; Feeling or Thinking; Good or Evil; Consciousness or Unconsciousness; Christianity or Hinduism. We split God in two and experience both sides of His/Her nature, which is Unity. Even when we as atheists explore the side which is No God, we are still exploring God in order to find the One.

It is when you go into these polarities in depth that an exploration takes place into unknown territory. You can go too far into extremes, and things begin to go out of shape, get out of proportion, and much suffering is the result. Yet without this suffering resulting from these experiences, real growth and learning, and real original creativity can't take place. Out of our suffering and mistakes new steps in the learning process come. For when in the afterlife state we have the opportunity to consider all that has happened in the life we have just lived, we can see how an injustice to the other side of the pole has been created. We may see how we have gone too far into the other extreme, and by that realisation we learn to exercise our gift of choice, and decide to journey into the other side in the next life. Experience is built up gradually from this swinging movement to and fro, in our attempt to find balance and justice.

As we grow and mature in our soul's journey, we will eventually be able to choose a lifetime where we bring about greater balance within that one lifetime. This is the karmic learning process which is the grounding, or school, of the soul for humanity. Karma is then speeded up, and as one can see, this is happening for many more people at the present time than has ever happened before. You will see this process increase in the next few years. We will no longer have to wait for death and afterlife to give us the perspective of greater awareness. Through your technology, your systems of communication on Earth are linking now, and you can have an immediate view of all the madness of collective hatred. Human scientific and technical development has made us one world.

I am moving on now and looking ahead to another major event in your life. The breakdown in health in which you undertook a living death in order to be rebuilt. You are rebuilding your body now: you have a new, a changed body structure. This has taken some time to accomplish. Normally it would have involved death and rebirth to a different set of parents, who would have been able to give you a new set of genetic instructions and new DNA. But this has been accomplished in one lifetime. M.E. and other new diseases such as AIDS are, in reality, processes whereby a new body structure for the whole of humanity can be forged. Many people have chosen to undergo these disease states as karmic experiences for humanity, as well as for themselves individually. Disease should not be seen always as negative, but a way by which we move forward collectively in our evolution.

We are all now in the process of receiving an increased input of Light. We are integrating light into our material structures. The new world will be peopled by a lighter race, but the accumulated experiences gathered by our soul in its journey from infancy through its many lifetimes, will have been gathered and transmuted by the body. All the elements of experience, of darkness and light, male and female, will have come together in order for a 'United Being of Light in whom the Dark Forever Shines', to be born. The new being will be the Child of that wholeness.

Perhaps that is enough for now. There is much more to say, and to clarify, but I will say it later if I may. Much love be with you.

BREAKING DOWN

Looking back from where I stand in the present moment, the decade which followed the birth of our beautiful daughter seems bleak and lonely, though it was also a period of growth and learning. I learned to be self-sufficient but without the loving support of a partner. I was alone for the first time, for although I loved my little daughter and she undoubtedly loved me, I was in sole charge, responsible for her welfare and for ensuring we had enough to survive.

I had shared a flat in South Kensington throughout the college years with four student artists: my two closest friends from Sheffield, Brian and Lena, and two young painters from St Albans, Richard Smith and Clare. Later I moved into a house in Chelsea once owned by the Victorian painter Alma Tadema. It was at that time owned by an elderly, disabled mathematician, who let his accommodation to a bevy of girls in return for keeping him company. The whole of the back garden had been converted by Alma Tadema into a studio, and several of us lived in that huge space in little enclaves. A trio of girls camped beneath the concert grand piano, two more slept on sofas round the stove at the far end, while others made their nests in alcoves and tiny anterooms. There were usually ten or more girls in the establishment at any one time. The mathematician was subject to bouts of suicidal depression and surrounded himself with what he called 'attractive young girls' to keep his spirits up. If this immediately seems to imply that he was an old roué, perish the thought! He was decidedly impotent and his legs were paralysed. But with the salary of a Dean of the Faculty of Science, and no one to spend it on, he liked to cut a figure in town by taking one of us out in turn, to a fashionable Soho restaurant and the theatre every night of the week.

These outings became such a routine for us 'girls', that the expensive high-life became just a boring duty. In a small way we were, for a time, the talk of the Chelsea Art Circuit, and it was probably hearing about this that led to Mahen contriving a meeting so that he might be introduced to 'the girls'. It was he who dubbed us alternatively, Doctor Cooke and the Cookies, or Doctor Crock and the Crockettes. We lived virtually rent-free in the studio, and in return we donned our most attractive gear and put on a little paint and powder and sailed off in the taxi with our elderly charge of an evening, to drink several brandies topped off with a Blue Curaçao or a Yellow Chartreuse.

When the relationship between Mahen and me became intense and serious, it seemed inappropriate to go on living with the girls and continuing my exotic duties, especially when I became pregnant. Mahen suggested that we should find somewhere to live together. At that precise moment, Lena, who had also had a child two weeks after a secret marriage to one of Britain's most influential painters, had moved to a house by the Regent's Canal in Islington and was looking for someone to look after her baby while she went out to teach. It seemed the ideal opportunity, as she was offering an empty flat for a small rent. It had been a wrench for me to leave the bevy of girlfriends and the Chelsea life, because I knew I would be putting that all behind me for good, and Islington seemed then, from my pad just off the King's Road, rather dull and unappealing; somewhere beyond the known Universe. But there was the lure of setting up a home, however lacking in basic essentials, with Mahen. It was my first experience of living as a twosome, and there was the close presence of my friend downstairs with her baby.

So I slipped the moorings from my old life in stages. The glamour still clung for a time, and also the dreams and hopes of an artist's life, which would continue with Mahen. In reality, those dreams were slipping away all too rapidly, but I was unable to see it. He was absent more and more. Out all day and coming home at night later and later. I would listen for sounds of his return in the darkness, not knowing if it were midnight or the early hours. But I didn't know how to read the signs. He was probably lying about his activities. Where he had been. With whom. But even then he would surprise me. Once, somewhere in the hours before dawn, he roused me from the empty cave of sleep I had sunk into, shaking me with an uncontainable excitement and tenderness. By the light from the street-lamp outside, he unwrapped a gramophone record he had carefully carried home, and set it on the wind-up player. In the grey light, feeling for the needle and the centre hole, his face, his eyes, creased up with the effort of containing his emotion. His hands danced now, as the strange, rich cadences began to flow; he crooned and burbled in his enthusiasm. 'You'll just die when you hear this. Listen to it. Listen while you're still half asleep, and then tell me that it's the most stunning, incredible music you have ever heard. I had to bring it for you. No one else I know will hear it like we do. I know you *say* you don't like Beethoven, but this is Beethoven like he never was. This is Beethoven ascended!' It was one of the late string quartets. I had never heard anything like it before. We lay in the dark, listening, and it was as if our souls communed.

Moments of beauty like this convinced me that in some special way we were connected in the true depth of our being. I still clung to the hope that things would come right. But the fact of the matter was, in the end, that he was not so much staying away from home increasingly often, as making the occasional visits to see me. Then he failed to appear at all, and I learned that he had gone to live in Paris. I was desolate and shocked. Gradually I had to undertake the business of making a life for Sandhya and myself alone. I adored her, and knew that her father was intensely proud of her too. He carried her photograph everywhere, and never lost the opportunity to bring it out of his pocket to show his acquaintances and boast about her. But that was as far as it went. All her needs had to be met by me, and there was no one for me to share a young mother's needs with, or meet the grief and loss which I felt.

Through that enforced situation, being a lone mother, I learned much, and I know I couldn't have done that if my life had been easier. If there had been a conventionally happy marriage with a kind and loving partner, we would no doubt have shared the pleasures and responsibilities of making a home. But as it was I learned to be father *and* mother to my child. Breadwinner and nurse, provider as well as nurturer. Bricklayer, plasterer, plumber, roof-repairer and gardener, as well as cook, cleaner, teacher and child-minder. There were, in that single parent role, to be many new relationships, new friendships, even romances. But always these were born out of neediness, out of pain, out of a desperate longing for reassurance and healing. And the more my despair and pain showed, the more men would shy away from commitment.

I came out of the Mahen experience with a deep sense of betrayal and rejection, and irrationally, the betrayal carried with it the feeling of unworthiness. A kind of guilt that I was somehow inadequate. Although there was anger at the way I had been treated, it was masked by the feeling that I was not good enough. My anger was impotent because it was ashamed. How could I allow myself to feel, never mind express, such an ignoble emotion? How could I admit to feelings of jealousy? Weren't we modern, broadminded, enlightened young people, above such base sentiments? So I attempted to deny them and squash them down.

The blossoms of love and trust that had begun to open were frosted. I felt betrayed. I had opened my heart in a way that had not been possible in previous relationships. With Andrea, I had been travelling on waves of romantic fantasy. With Brian, a much more real and truly felt relationship, I had nevertheless been the object of his youthful sexual desires. I often felt aroused in his presence, yet because of his demanding need to copulate at all costs, I felt used and violated. I could not have explained, even to myself, what it was that felt violated, because that feminine sexual being hadn't had the chance to become conscious. The gentle, subtle eroticism which, when it is given space, flowers into strong, colourful passion, had been overwhelmed by the onslaught of lust.

For some fateful reason I had found something in Mahen, and not in Brian, which called that being out. I had opened my inner self to him and found response. Felt, for a moment, a shimmering surge of beauty burst in my body, and a sensation like one of those Japanese paper flowers that you drop in water. A thirsty and dehydrated pellet, transformed into a fragile but exotic bloom by the new element it suddenly finds itself in. As it burgeoned I greeted it with delight. Something in Mahen responded, and for a while two tender beings danced together. Then the spell was broken. For him it had been an interlude and held no place in his world of stark reality. Both the inner child we had discovered within ourselves, and the baby in the outer world, were now highly inconvenient. The prospect of having to nurture and take personal responsibility for either of these tender infants was out of the question.

Not that he didn't make every attempt to arrange affairs honourably, but it was always clear that he could never allow domestic coils to entrap him. We stayed together for the first year of our daughter's life, but things grew increasingly acrimonious. Her arrival might have been an event which added richness and joy to our lives, but instead he withdrew and distanced himself from her. I felt his rejection of her even more keenly than his treatment of me. This child, whose moment of creation we had shared with such wonder and tenderness, was now his reason for taking off.

Oh! A.Z., you talk of the child of the union symbolising all those wonderful things, Unity, Wholeness, Peace, which at one level she did. When I discovered the meaning of the name 'Sandhya', it felt as if I had touched upon a mystery I could hardly grasp. Intimations of another reality known to a higher, deeper self which foreshadowed an inner marriage between the Yin and the Yang; the darkness and the light within me. All of this I was yet to discover at some point in the future. I was only aware at the time of the wonder of the lovely child I had brought into the world, and the difficulties that it had thrown up. Her birth and the near-death experience had been an important milestone in my spiritual development. But the actual reality, the every day, down to earth level, was where I had to live. It was there I had to face the stark reality of making ends meet. All those fair and honourable arrangements for her welfare which Mahen started out with, came to nothing. Instead he left me with his debts, and I gritted my teeth and floundered around looking for ways to cope. What assets did I have? What training for life? No qualifications, no money in the bank, no stamps on my card.

On top of this, something had happened during the birth. Although that near-death experience had been illuminating in the way it lifted my understanding of life onto a new plane, physically I emerged from it shaken, weak and thin. The tears I had shed and shared with the midwife never really dried up. Postnatal blues developed into a persistent state of depression which came and went. I lost the buoyancy and resilience I once had, and a dark, dense cloud seemed to float above me, sapping my energy and bearing down on me. In my dreams I would be climbing up the mountain, once more reaching for a ledge that would bring me within reach of the top, only the burden on my back prevented me from pulling myself upwards. Always my strength was insufficient for the task ahead.

One of the ways in which Mahen had been helpful before he went, was by beginning to search for a suitable house. We had looked at possible ways for me to have a place to live with Sandhya, and also something that would provide a source of income. Considering that I was unqualified for a well-paid job, it didn't seem realistic that I could earn enough to cover a mortgage and successfully bring up a child at the same time. The theoretical solution we arrived at was to buy one of those old, rundown Islington houses, which were still reasonably cheap in 1960. But where was the money to come from? Mahen's mother had already cut him off when she heard of his goings on in London, so there was nothing for it but to turn to my parents. Difficult though that was, because of their strong disapproval and the pain we had caused them by our relationship, we decided to swallow our pride and ask them for help.

The nettle grasped, we took the train to Sheffield, knowing we would have to face a barrage of recriminations, and tears, which were harder to bear. But after putting our case to them, my father came to my rescue in the end, mainly for the sake of Sandhya, who he loved dearly from the day of her birth. He promised to give me the money to buy a house large enough to be divided into flats. This would hopefully provide a safe home for her, a studio for me, and a source of income from renting out the other flats. When the moment came after a long search and I found the house I felt was suitable, I had quite a tussle with my father. In spite of his generosity, he firmly clung onto the purse strings and wanted to dictate to me who I should have as tenants. He tried long and hard to persuade me to chose a house in a respectable suburb, and not the run down Georgian terraces of the then unfashionable Islington, which attracted me because of their elegant proportions.

Eighteen months after Sandhya was born and six months after Mahen had disappeared, we bought a five-storey house for a little over £4000. Although it sustained me, more or less, over the next decade or so, by providing an income from a motley collection of tenants, it also drained my energies. It towered over me and dragged me down, as much as it sheltered me. Its roof leaked constantly, and endless amounts of cash were needed to pour into its repair. The drains were faulty, its plumbing and wiring, installed by the previous owner, a mad Greek, were lethal, and wound through the interstices of walls and under floorboards, like a writhing clutch of malicious giant worms, leaking and sparking. There was woodworm and dry rot in the fabric and I was endlessly putting to use my mountaineering skills, clambering over the slippery, slate precipice of the roof, five storeys high, with buckets of hot tar, or up ladders, painting, spraying and plastering because the rents didn't cover paying the extortionate rates which local builders demanded.

The small back garden was dominated by two huge elm trees under whose shade *nothing* would grow. Their roots, too close to the surface, sucked every bit of goodness out of the earth, and very little sunshine ever got in through the canopy. I dug and I fertilised, planted and despaired. All my plants died. I shouldn't give the impression that our life was nothing but gloom and disaster. Far from it. The story is like a two sided coin, one side golden, bright and shiny, and the other side dark. But the dark side grew to be so dominant that it overpowered me in the end, and broke me down. Somehow this house and garden became a symbol. It seemed to put into a nutshell the psychologically disempowering situation that I succumbed to. Seeing my efforts to make a flourishing garden in spite of the impoverished soil, friends came to help. We constructed compost heaps and filled them with plant matter and leaves, which we gathered from the local parks, but the trees were too strong for us and gobbled up the nourishment and closed their branches against the sun, and our plants struggled and our efforts wilted beneath them.

The house and garden, in a Thurberesque sort of way, developed a life of its own. It became an image which preyed upon me. Frequent dreams of this towering house, decaying and crumbling, and the looming trees sucking out the virtue from the earth, seemed to sum up my situation. However much money, energy or love was poured into their maintenance, and quite a lot of love was poured in, the end effect was that they demanded more and more. I struggled to earn money from my sculpture to replenish the coffers, I considered teaching jobs, but undermined myself by feeling that I had nothing worthwhile to teach. This probably stemmed from the 'bout of doubt' which had overtaken me in my second year at college, and the feeling that I was out of step with the new art movements of the late 60's and 70's.

My passions at that time were still involved with figures that resonated to nature: organic form, plants or animals, and all of that had gone out of fashion. Instead of feeling happy and fulfilled in the work I was doing, as I had in the early days of Art School, I experimented with other forms which didn't spring truly from my soul, but I was deceiving myself. I should have learned that lesson from the time in Rome when I also tried to change myself to fit in with something foreign to my nature.

The challenges of teaching scared me too much, and although I went for a few interviews for art school posts, in my imagination I saw myself being put in charge, not of compliant, respectful, mature students eager to learn from me, but of gangs of rebellious, anarchic and hostile adolescents, calling my aesthetic beliefs into question. So I looked elsewhere for work, only to find myself competing with the poorest women in the neighbourhood for cleaning, washing up or homeworking, or addressing envelopes for a penny a hundred. I felt, probably like them, a victim of society; an exploited, powerless failure.

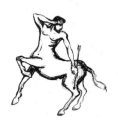

THROUGH A GLASS DARKLY

(and a conversation with A.Z.)

Late at night a stranger knocks at your door. In Crete he is called the unknown god. There, all doors and hearts are opened to him. The finest supper is prepared in his honour and he is invited to sleep between the softest sheets. What if this stranger is an aspect of our self? Can we draw him also into the light of our compassion?

When I set out to write this story, I didn't know where it would lead, how far I would go or what I would uncover. Inevitably, when you undertake a journey into your life, there will be areas which are easier to enter: positive places which you can enjoy exploring again because they affirm you in some way. Then there will be more difficult areas that you don't so easily want to go into. You may have shut the door on them because behind the door is pain and darkness and shame. You tell yourself you shouldn't reopen old wounds. But unless old wounds are truly healed they are not finished with. Let in the light of the heart. Compassion. Loving the dark stranger who is yourself, accepting and forgiving, this is the most truly healing act. When you have learned to love yourself, *then* you can love your neighbour and love the world.

But these things cannot be rushed. If we push too fiercely on a closed door, we may only do more damage. Resistances may be in place for a good reason, and defences erected because that was the only way to survive at the time. Wisdom tells us to go gently, with a light touch, and the locked doors will yield and reveal the things we have hidden away, in their own good time, when we are ready.

When I approached this point in my life-review, I felt a sense of apprehension. The door was firmly closed, and I didn't want to open it in case all manner of black-winged creatures came screeching out. But I knew the time had come. Being ready didn't necessarily mean that it would be painless, but, I thought, if I can bear to touch it, hold out my hand and try to welcome and accept it, then maybe a new healing can begin.

So I came to the door which was shut. It seemed black and forbidding. I tentatively tapped upon it and it began to creak open on its rusty hinges just a little bit, and there seemed to be a sigh and a breath of air; a chink of light. I began to wonder why I had been so afraid after all, as the first pictures to emerge were happy. Undertakings well completed, new relationships developed and nurtured, and above all, the sunshine years of my little daughter growing up. This surprised me. There was a golden side of the coin after all. By trying to close out the pain of the past, I had shut out so much else.

Having been an only child myself, and without much in the way of maternal leanings, I had little experience of children. So Sandhya's babyhood was a revelation to me. Soon we were sharing the usual childhood joys of park and beach. We paddled and see-sawed, made sand-castles and ate ice-creams. We painted our faces and dressed up. I was discovering an important part of myself; reliving my own childhood.

Because I tended to be rather shy and found it hard to initiate friendships, I might have gone on for years without getting to know anyone. But I discovered that a child is the passport into a club of aficionados. When I was twelve I had a dog which was the love of my life. Maybe because I was an only child, he took the place of brothers and sisters for me. I would even get up in the middle of the night and creep down to the kitchen, sit on the floor in the dark and talk to him. We would go everywhere and do everything together, and on our walks around the houses or across the park, people would stop without ceremony to speak to us. Now I found when I was out with Sandhya in the pram, or on the bus, that inevitably someone would start up a conversation preluded by, 'Oh! What a lovely baby.' She had an astonishingly sweet nature, which seemed to captivate strangers and friends alike.

The first three years of her life, I decided, I would devote to giving her a good grounding and sense of security, but after that I would try to get back to my work again. I had imagined myself, in those anxious days before her birth, wielding hammer and chisel, pieces flying in all directions across the studio floor, while a plaster covered baby crawled about my feet. But by the time reality dawned, I found that I had become besottedly absorbed in the day by day stages of her development, and filled with maternal pride. So the decision to suspend my sculpture was not too difficult. By three years she was eager to start nursery school, and I remember her delight, on the first day, when she was given her own possessions with a picture to identify them instead of her name. A little cup and plate, a place to hang her coat, and wonder of wonders, a little bed for the afternoon rest. She enjoyed it so much it was hard to get her to come home. She graduated to the infants class two years later without any problem.

Like-minded people tend to congregate together, and this Cannonbury school had attracted newcomers who had been drawn to this part of London for similar reasons to myself, as well as the old established Islington families. I think we were resented by some, who saw this influx as a middle class invasion, but the grand terrace houses were originally built for the middle-class. There have always been groups of people moving in and out, and at that time, in the Sixties, our area was an exciting melting pot. Young artists, writers, architects, craftsmen, researchers, musicians, politicians, as well as stray hippies and drop-outs, all came to be a part of the local community. They fused together with the local Islington population of native Londoners, Greek and Turkish Cypriots, Irish, West Indian – the lot – every shape and colour, creating a vibrant and stimulating mix.

It wasn't long before Sandhya and I had become woven into that community, and acquired a strong and supportive group of friends. Far from being that bleak and foreign place which it had seemed before I went to live there, I found Islington enriching. It changed me; I was broadening, maturing, in the alchemy of the melting pot. I may well have gravitated towards more responsible and down-to-earth people if I had stayed in Chelsea, but there I was still ensnared by the glamour of a gay and carefree artist's life. Through becoming a parent and a house-holder in Islington, I began to be aware of something lacking in myself, and I set about trying to do something about it. I began to develop a so-cial conscience or, rather, a consciousness of my relationship to the community. When actions needed to be taken, or people needed to be defended, then I would have to stand up and be counted, rather than have the luxury, as I had done in the past, of holding strong views about social injustice, but never putting them into action. I suppose I became more visible as a personality. I put my head above the parapet, and discovered that visibility invites attack.

It also invites support.

I was gathering a group of interesting friends. There were the O'Connors: the father was a graduate engineer and there were four energetic and forever scrapping children. Marthy, their mother, was a warm, gregarious woman who held court in her ever open house just around the corner, and through her I met many sculptors, painters and writers who had newly arrived in the area. The doors of the O'Connor establishment were never locked and friends were encouraged to drop in at any time, so that an endless troop of us were to be seen going in and out at all hours, refreshed by cups of tea and sympathy. This is probably why, one after-noon, when two strange men walked in and exited with several family possessions in their arms, no one realised they were witnessing a burglary.

Lucien Freud's family lived close by and we played in their garden with their two children, Rosy and Alexander, and ate home-made marmalade cake. A few doors away was another painter, Sue D, who soon became a close friend. Her husband was a jazz musician and their house, like Marthy's, was a community meeting place. Sue, unlike Marthy, had a strong political outlook, and this led to me introducing one of Mahen's old Sri Lankan cronies to her when she was looking for a tenant. Several of his friends then joined him and they would spend their nights loudly propounding the rival merits of Che Guevara or Uncle Ho's revolutionary methods. This mixture of smoking left wing political arguments and improvised jam sessions, resulted in some red-hot vibrations issuing from the walls of this particular house late into the night.

Sue's husband was very fond of Sandhya, and often took her along with his two children on adventurous expeditions. She was very popular and was never without offers to spend nights, weekends, or even weeks away with various families. A particularly close friend at school was Kay, and I was quite friendly with Kay's mother. She lived with her man friend and another woman in a ménage à trois, also presiding over a 'come and go as you please' household where there was opportunity to get to know a medley of interestingly complex and individual people. Kay's mother was, in the Sixties, one of the forerunners of Women's Lib, and she was also actively involved in socialist causes. She organised a support movement for the miners who were holding a strike at the time, collecting food and money for their families.

For a good few years Sandhya's friendship with Kay was one which meant a lot to both girls. She was able to develop her independence and spirit as she was growing up. They went on demonstrations together with Kay's mother and her political friends, they joined the local boat club run for all the kids who lived by the Regent's Canal and learned to survive being upturned in the water, and they went to the Isle of Wight together and stayed with Kay's grandmother at her country estate, and sampled raspberries fresh picked from the kitchen garden by the butler.

Maybe though, one of the most important figures in Sandhya's life, *and* in my own, was Carl. Theoretically, I knew how valuable having older male friends would be for Sandhya in the absence of her father, but these friendships came about quite by chance and just seemed to grow naturally, and I met this family within a few weeks of her birth. At first it was Carl's wife, Emma, who shepherded me through the crucial early days, when all was new to me in the art of babycare. She introduced me to the invaluable Dr Benjamin Spock and supported me with humour and practical advice.

She also introduced me to a wonderful local GP who was, a year or two later, to give me, freely, an hour of his time once a week. This developed into valuable therapeutic counselling during the time when I became severely depressed. If I don't say more about him, it is because there is too much to say. He is a remarkable and unsung man who has counselled and supported many, including survivors of the Nazi concentration camps, and done so out of a generous heart, and without publicity.

As for Carl himself, I saw him only infrequently at first as he dropped in, bushed, after work, to say hello to Emma and the kids, before going up to his den to crash out. It was only gradually, over the years, that a deep friendship grew up between us. I will return to Carl and Emma again later.

* * *

We gave our energy and enthusiasm to life in the city and received much in return. But this positive side began to give way to the darker elements of conflict and aggression which seemed to be gaining ground all around. To me, London as a whole was becoming more angry, crooked and threatening day by day. The pace of life grew faster and people became dishonest, mean, mistrustful. The state of community which I had felt a part of once, was fast becoming a state of war. People became sharper and tougher. The attitude was, you have to give as hard as you get, in order to survive, and, to my dismay, I saw more and more people going along with that.

It was a dilemma. Was I going to have to learn to be ruthless and hard skinned in order not to go under? Gradually, I was putting up fences – literally! All round my property they went up, and bars at the windows, to keep out the encroachment of unruly neighbourhood children left to their own devices by fathers and mothers out all day earning a living as best they could, and out all evening drowning their sorrows. All the adjoining gardens became a rat-run and an adventure playground for the untended kids who swarmed over the walls, threw stones at the windows, set fires, took pot-shots at cats, and generally created mayhem. There were constant break-ins, or drunken husband and wife punch-ups in the street at night, and one was constantly on the watch for the 'cowboys' and swindlers out to take you for a ride. Suddenly, it had turned from a stimulating and supportive community into a threatening one. Some of my friends were skilled at surviving in these conditions and still remaining decent at heart, but I felt vulnerable and corroded by its poison.

Alone with my dilemma, I brooded in the house at night. Insecure and without support, I couldn't see where this life was leading. Day by day my health was deteriorating, and my income was dwindling, until I only had three pounds a week to live on. Insecurity and anxiety ate away at me and I was overcome by a severe depression, which caused me, after I had taken Sandhya to school in the morning, to come back to my basement room, lock myself in, and cover myself up with the bedclothes. I would lie there for hours trying to blot out the pain and desolation and the sense of utter helplessness and hopelessness. The problems in the outer world were only a small part of it. There was a chasm of despair inside: a hollow self-devouring emptiness which had sucked out all the life-spirit which had once flowed through my veins.

When I attempt to write about these times now, Astrazzurra, my guiding star, try as I will, the picture becomes too confused and cloudy. It's like looking into a dark pool, and I can't see clearly any more.

It was an experience in which you found yourself being washed away. You lost your footing and felt out of your depth. You were overwhelmed by a tidal wave of circumstances, which were more powerful than the power you had within yourself to cope. So there was a deficit – a power imbalance.

Your longings for a male partner who would support you was an inner cry for balance. It was a situation which needed the masculine as well as the feminine qualities. Yet you needed them at the physical level: muscle power in great quantities, and you tried to supply that out of your own strength. It needed cooperation and commitment. You had a certain amount of cooperation but the commitment was lacking. There was help, but it was insufficient.

Where there is harmony of purpose, and a recognition and respect for the qualities which each person can give to the whole, then in a marriage or community you have an organic complex which nurtures and strengthens the members. This is a wide subject, but it reflects the issues we touched on before, of the Ideal City based on sacred geometric structures. A marriage and a family have a sacred structure: a wonderful singing, resounding harmony which feeds and respects the diversity of the individuals who make it up. A sacred community works in the same way, embracing families and individuals. Each contributes her or his gifts, and in return receives sustenance.

This is the ideal, but what we have at the moment in society is far from the ideal. When I say sacred, I am not meaning under the religious authority of a church. Sacred is when the note given off sounds beautiful. If you have a crystal glass vase of high quality and craftsmanship, it 'sings' a sweet and perfect sound when you strike it. Sacred marriage and sacred community work towards achieving that beauty of sound. But the sounds in our cities and in our families in most cases at present, are very jarring and clashing.

That is a wonderful vision, A.Z., but so very far from the situation I found myself in. I was certainly in need of a committed friend and support through these times, but in those first years I had to turn to society's system for help. The officials and the bureaucrats who dole out money along with judgements and prejudices.

You went out into the world and the World responded in its way.

I tried to earn my keep, but found that I could get only the most menial and ridiculously underpaid jobs.

Women's work was still greatly undervalued and women's role was undervalued. You were suddenly flung into a role you hadn't prepared for. You found yourself in a situation which you had neither foreseen nor planned. From the start, Mahen had foreseen what having a child would entail for him and knew he couldn't cope with it. But you took responsibility upon yourself, as mothers are wont to do. Your first priority was to the child, and your career came second. You felt a strong loyalty to your art and pursued your career with a struggle, but felt so dispirited and drained by events that your creativity suffered.

There is a great fountain or well-spring which is the source of our creativity. It is situated near the Sacral, or Abdomen, Chakra in the belly. That source must be nurtured and fed, given a strong foundation in early life and sustained thereafter. You were let down in your early life by your mother. The mother is so important. The Great Mother within us is the nurturer of our creativity. She is the source of this energy: the God-Self energy. The Motherhood of God is the source from which we draw our life force.

If the earthly mother is insufficient and fails to nurture the source within her child, then we need to become that mother to ourselves; loving ourselves unconditionally. If things have gone badly for us, then this can't happen until we are at a place in life where there is a certain degree of security, where we can rest, recuperate and begin to repair the damage.

The course of your life was mapped out beforehand, and the valley of the shadow which you entered was known to you before your birth. You had chosen to enter it and as you came into life you wavered, knowing what troubles were ahead of you. The first pages of your story intimate your reluctance to come down to Earth. Strange, was it not, that the midwife you depict there, standing in the patch of sunlight at the time of your birth, was a reflection of the midwife who called you back again when Sandhya was born? How much you wanted to escape again to those wonderful Elysian Fields. Who could blame you? But again you chose to come back and take care of a new life.

This is courage. You had great courage to persist in your task. You could have said no, but you went on with your assignment. There is far more to all of this than you are aware of right now, but we won't go into complications. You came back to balance relationships forged in previous lives – Mahen, Brian, Andrea – your lives have interwoven down the ages many times. I have been with you also, and have lived with you in the past.

So, you were thrown out into the world – expelled from the security of the garden of Eden, if you like, where you had walked as an art student, and now were experiencing the World's judgement! The Source, the well-spring of creative flow, and the favour and fortune which you had known, had begun to dry up. Instead you experienced deprivation, condemnation, loneliness and depression, and this deepened into exhaustion.

In the disease M.E. you experienced the wasting away of all the body's systems. Your health was undermined, and you became a target for micro-organisms to enter. The fact that you decided to struggle bravely on, only debilitated you further. At the same time you were subject to an onslaught of thought forces. People all around you were telling you to pull yourself together when you had no resources left to draw upon, so that your attempt to do as they were demanding depleted even further your substances, and weakened your basic fabric. But still it went on. The body always tries to mend itself, it is a natural spontaneous intelligence. Yet every time it responded intelligently, demands were put upon it before it could regain its strength. People told you that your condition was 'all in the mind', implying that what you knew about yourself was a lie.

Yes. This is all part of the familiar story of these dark years. Yet I am poised at the edge of it looking into it, and it still feels as if I'm at the edge of a dark pool and I am fearing to go further in. There are things in there still too difficult to handle. I can see where it continues on the other side, strangely enough. The horrors of the illness itself are much clearer, but there seems to be a gap just here, and I can't cross it. Help me to go on. Tell me what it is I can't see.

I'll help you, but I can't do the seeing for you. Just ask your own wisdom and intuition for clearer vision. Let's stand there together in an open receptive meditative state, on the edge of the pool as it were, and see what comes.

(After a while, a picture emerges.)

I am standing out in the road and it is Maytime, or perhaps June. I am feeling good about myself. I've taken myself in hand ... going to start a cleansing diet ... made an appointment for a Nature Cure Clinic and I'm feeling confident that I can reverse the decline in my health. The fatigue that has been plaguing me, the aches and pains in my muscles, and the trouble in my guts, the sickness and diarrhoea, which have become a chronic problem. I'm feeling both confident and determined on this bright, spring day.

Maggie, our neighbour, is getting out of her van, and seems to be making a beeline for me. She is a bit of a moaner, deceitful and something of a gossip and a troublemaker, and I don't particularly want to have a conversation with her right now. But it is too late! I can't escape. She is making clear tracks for me.

'I've got some news for you,' she says straight out. 'Your friend Carl is dead. They found him this morning. He's committed suicide.'

And all I could think of saying, was – You bitch! Fancy coming out with a stupid story like that! Do you expect me to be taken in by it? How typical to be making a joke of something like that.

I don't say any of this out loud, because her words are exploding in my head and my mouth opens in shock. One part of me is believing what she is saying, because it discerns right away that it is *true* – while another, slower part, reacts in unspoken, inner words, disbelieving. For a moment the two parts are in conflict, fighting against each other, and then I *know* which part is perceiving the truth. *Carl is dead*, and it is as if part of me has quit also, right at that moment. Part of me has died.

We were very close, Carl and I. His wife Emma – warm, good looking, intelligent Emma, who had so befriended me just after Sandhya was born – now had a research job with the BBC, and their lives were growing more and more apart. I had given Carl the spare bed in my studio and he had been living there for a couple of months. Emma was incredibly broadminded about sexual freedom in marriage, but there was no love affair going on between her husband and me. No romantic or sexual attachment between us. He just needed a place to be for a while to sort things out. But in the last year or two Carl and I had got to know each other well. We shared our lives, our innermost thoughts and outer problems, and we had shared a great deal of fun. We had outings together, with Sandhya and Carl's two children, and other assorted kids from the neighbourhood. He was tall and fair and handsome, full of energy and ideas, and we had enjoyed being part of the lively community life of Islington in the Sixties. Together with the children we had indulged in 'child's play': swimming, expeditions, escapades, theatre club, carnivals, fireworks, music-making, holidays, parties. We discovered that, participating in the child's world with our input of enthusiasm, fun and creative ideas, we had given a new lease of life to our own world.

But as well as the fun and games, we shared with each other our spiritual searching, our challenges and our problems. We were open to each other's pains and rejections, and to the consequences of our hideous mistakes. He had become an alcoholic over the years as his marriage became more shaky. Perhaps it was the other way round! But during a particularly rough patch a few years before, when he had been temporarily kicked out of the matrimonial home, he had gone on a binge and ended up at a party. In a wild attempt to get away from the tensions and conflicts at home, he was throwing himself into the festive mood, unaware that Emma had been invited to the same party. They suddenly came face to face. Carl spun round and fled the scene in panic, jumped into his car and stepped hard on the accelerator. A thirteen year old girl had just stepped into the road and was part way across. He hit her and she died instantly. He was shocked and devastated: his own daughter was about the same age, and he loved all children.

He was still coming to terms with this disaster. He had stuck to his vow never to drink again, and since leaving prison he had committed himself to prison visiting. His present job was warden at a halfway house for newly released, homeless, alcoholic prisoners. He was an intelligent, sensitive and capable man, and in the past I'd felt a bit overawed by the fact that he had a high-powered responsible job with the Commonwealth Office, dealing on a daily basis with foreign delegations. However, on many levels we were alike, and I saw several parallels in our lives, but on this level I had felt out of my depth. I would never have had the confidence to mingle with the sort of people he came in contact with in his previous job. Apart from that, we might be described as soul mates. Our spiritual searching, the sharing of our depths and despairs, our disagreeing, arguing, laughing and co-rejoicing was a shared journey. But until the shock of his death, I didn't recognise how much I identified with him.

This is interesting. You have touched on something here, haven't you? Carl comes up as a subject for your story, but you don't like where it is leading. You admitted, that is, let in, the shock which Maggie caused when she told you of his death, and you now see it more clearly as a cause of the onset of the M.E. In his suicide you recognise your own suicide. Part of you committed suicide. I don't like that term, 'committed' it carries judgement, but however...   You see yourself in his struggle, and in his failure you saw no option but to fail yourself. Because, at that time, you thought that your abilities to succeed and overcome your problems were inferior to his.

You saw him as courageous in the face of great difficulties. More courageous than you. More talents, more competence. Yet, he was overcome and he killed himself. How could you then go on? Yet you wanted to go on. It wasn't your way to cop out, and because he had copped out, you felt let down. Now you were alone.

You can see how his 'opt-out strategy' undermined your confidence in your ability to survive and succeed, to such an extent that the part of you that decided to go on (as opposed to the part of you that wanted to opt out also) was weakened and depleted of energy. Your belief that you had less chance of survival than him, caused your depletion. You had measured yourself against him and found yourself wanting. You had, or you believed you had, no resources to draw on, because you didn't believe there were any resources available to you.

The fact that you went on in this condition, weakened and depleted in mind and body, meant that the organisms were able to invade and deal a devastating blow. You opened yourself up to them, and they came in.

In time, over the next few years, your system was broken down until everything was withdrawn, and you became totally dependent. You will tell that part of the story soon. In some ways this is an adventure story, though you would be the first to say, 'No thanks! Who would choose to suffer like that as an adventure?' But many do. Think of those who go to the Poles and end up frozen skin and bones. They expect everyone to applaud them for their endurance and courage. Some choose to go to the highest mountain top without oxygen or Sherpas – others trek the dry and blistering deserts, or sit on the top of a pole* in the wilderness and waste away, and the World acclaims them as saints. Maybe they should call them fools! But they hit the headlines, and become noted, even famous for their extraordinary suffering which they brought upon themselves. What is the difference?

You chose to go to extremes and explore the depths of yourself in order to discover the resources which you failed to believe in at first. You dis-

---

* Again, I was rather slow. I had read this passage over several times before it dawned on me that A.Z. was using language in rather a poetical, three dimensional way once again. On page 152 he had commented on 'going to the poles', in another context. But now I suddenly saw just how it applied to me.

covered the Universal Power – the power of miracle, within yourself. It was always there, and along with it are an infinite variety of creative possibilities for you yet to discover. Who would believe it? No one it seems believes it of themselves, yet it is there. It is so. You have only touched on the tip of it and for that you paid a great price, because you believed you had to pay the price of suffering. Nothing so joyful and wonderful could be had for free.

So you set out on an adventure, a quest, like the mythological heroes and saints of old, going through trials and tribulations before being granted the golden prize. You are taking part in Humanity's story, but it is a story that is about to open a new chapter. Suffering must now be left behind as a way, or path, to the Golden Dawn.

But let's carry on in the meantime with your story. The adventure of suffering that you set out on, and the tale of how you eventually discovered the power of Healing, out of the experience of Woundedness and Pain.*

I had planned a health campaign. I was starting a five-day fast the following day. Carl's death had dealt me a blow, but my life would go on as planned. I completed the first three days without food and was amazed to find that, although I was a little weak and light-headed, I really felt better. I had clear skin and eyes, a different quality of energy, and in addition I was composed and relaxed. Although, because of the lower energy levels it was difficult to manage the shopping and cooking, the journeys on foot to school and back, as well as fitting in my own work; I just did everything more slowly. On the fourth day of the regime I was allowed to eat my first meal of fruit, and the orange I had for breakfast tasted as if it had come from the Garden of Paradise. Then I had a mixture of oranges, apricots and cherries for lunch, and more of the same for supper.

---

* My story illustrates one scenario which led to ill health, but I think many people fail to understand that *all disease*, not just for me – not just for M.E., but for everyone – is an indication of imbalance.

Dis-comfort, dis-ease, is a message from your body telling you that something is needing attention. When you ignore or misinterpret this message the signals get louder. It may be a physical need you are ignoring, or an emotional, mental or spiritual need, but if you haven't understand the message over a long period of time (because it is very likely that the messages started to arrive in early childhood,) then the body itself will begin to develop more serious dysfunctions. It has tried to communicate in its own wise way by speaking 'body language', providing you with a symptom which symbolises its dis-ease, but if these messages have gone unheard, more serious and intractable conditions may set in which are harder to heal.

What are your legs telling you? Your heart, stomach, liver? Your throat, your head, your arms and hands?

I went to bed feeling well pleased with myself and delighted by the noticeable improvement in my condition. I was looking forward to the following day when I could have a mixture of raw vegetables and salads. Then the fast would be over and I could eat normally again.

Somewhere in the middle of the night I woke up burning with fever, and was aware of intense pain in my feet. My whole body was red-hot. What on earth was happening? I had heard of a healing crisis, was this it? I was sweating; maybe this was the body ridding itself of poisons. But alarmingly, the pains in my feet, already intense, began to creep up my legs: up my ankles, calves, into the knee joints, then up into my thighs and hip joints. The left side became so painful I hardly knew what to do with myself. Then it was everywhere. In my neck, head, chest and arms. My body was wracked and shaking with the pain. It came in waves and spasms, and I was gasping, helpless and hardly able to move.

At last, exhausted, I must have fallen asleep, for it was now daylight. I was more than alarmed, I was scared. If this was a healing crisis, it was more than I had bargained for. I couldn't cope with it and I must ring the doctor. He would be none too pleased, since I had taken things into my own hands when I contacted the Nature Cure Clinic and decided on this campaign. I feared he would be scathing and disapproving. Yet I had to get help. I sat up weakly, put my feet on the floor, and made to get up. But as I put my weight onto my feet, my legs gave way. All strength had gone, and I had to crawl into the next room where the telephone was and haul myself up on the chair to make the call.

Here began a long, long nightmare and tale of horror. Visits to doctors, hospitals, examinations, tests, which at the end of the day (and it was a very long day indeed, a day which lengthened into years) resulted in me being labelled unstable, neurotic, emotionally labile, an attention seeker, a time waster, a hysteric, and every label the medical profession could throw at me to cover up the fact that they didn't know or understand the reason for my illness. Rather than admit that they didn't know, as that would have weakened their authority and the air of omniscience they sought to maintain, they resorted to projecting onto me, the patient, all the weaknesses and fallibilities of character that they could dredge up.

SIX

DESCENT

Toll the bell
Cannot tell
How she fell
Down the well

Bell's told
Couldn't hold
Feel the cold

Cold as hell she fell.

Cold as clay
Clam as toad
Dropping, dropping,
Giving way.
Giving way,
Cannot hold
Where's the stop?

Drop. Drop.

Heart's wings
Beating hard
Beating hard

Against the fall.
Battering, clutching,
Scrapes the wall.
Fighting hard
The downward flight,
Plummets down
The shaft of night.

Hands pressed
Heart to still.
Stillness crying
What of will?
Can she fill
This All-Alone:
This empty throne
Turned to stone?

Petrifying;
Peter's crying;
Rock denying.
Let my cry ....
Echo, echo.
Ecce Homo.

Esmé Ellis 1985

BEGINNING THE DESCENT

I feel no enthusiasm whatsoever for reopening this chapter of my life. I have a natural distaste for dwelling on details of illness, either my own or anyone else's. But it must be told, and in as much detail as I can muster, otherwise what followed, the extraordinary events of spiritual dimensional healing and the guidance which went alongside that healing, will not be fully understood.

M.E. is becoming widely recognised nowadays, though not every doctor accepts its reality still. When it first afflicted me it was virtually unknown, in the sense that there was no name or label for it, though those who had it knew all about it. When I called my doctor the morning after that awful night in 1969, and awoke to find I couldn't stand up, he came round promptly. It was obvious that I was in a bad way, for as well as the shock of losing the use of my lower limbs, I had a high fever and was very shaky. So he quickly arranged for me to go into the out-patient's clinic at the Rheumatology Department of the Royal Free Hospital. There was something ironic in this, since there had been an outbreak of M.E. there ten or fifteen years previously, when almost three hundred nurses and doctors and other staff had mysteriously gone down with the disease. But since the scientists in the laboratories had been unable to pinpoint a causal agent, virus or whatever, it was decided that the cause was mass hysteria. However, further outbreaks occurred from time to time in different locations both in this country and around the world, and the name 'Royal Free Disease' was attached to it for a time. But because it was an embarrassment to the profession to acknowledge that a group of their own kind had succumbed to what they had designated a hysterical disease, they probably tried to forget about it and pretend the whole thing had never happened.

It certainly didn't ring any bells with the young doctor who examined me and put me through a whole battery of tests. The first thing they looked for were signs of osteomyelitis and rheumatic fever. That was followed up by tests for several out of the way possibilities, including a rare sheep disease, and I must say they were very thorough. But in the end, after many difficult trips to the hospital (for I had to learn to cope

176

with this sudden inability to walk) their conclusion was that I must be suffering from a 'mild muscular rheumatism.'

If this was mild, I thought, then heaven help me if something more severe struck. I couldn't seem to get across to anyone the severity of the pain, nor the great difficulty I was suddenly having in standing up or attempting to walk. They obviously concluded it was psychosomatic. I either had to accept their diagnosis, which to me was hopelessly insufficient, or find some way to make them understand. But the more I tried, the more they saw me as a neurotically disturbed patient constructing a fantasy illness out of a mild disease. And the more they saw me in *this* role, the less patience they had with my predicament.

To give them their due, it is a very difficult disease to recognise: no two people experience it in the same way. It can occasionally strike in epidemic form, but more often it hits people individually. Then again, some are affected only slightly and for a short time, whilst others, like myself, can experience a very severe form, and the disabling and debilitating symptoms can go on for many years. But there are a few main symptoms which are common to all cases and are clinically described as: extreme weakness or profound fatigue, extreme malaise with acute tenderness in some muscles, impairment of memory and difficulty in finding the right word and in completing a sentence, pallor and coldness of extremities. Plus a pattern of relapse and recovery. The relapses, more often than not, are brought on by attempting physical or even mental activity too soon while still in the infectious state.

Since the objective reality of the disease was denied or not known, when I sought attention, pressure was put on me to ignore what was taking place in my body, and strive to carry on as usual. Not only that, but I was made to feel that I was being weak and spineless, and indulging in pathological fantasy to boot. So I drove myself on when I should have given myself permission to recover.

For two years I struggled with the tasks of everyday living, and found myself having to use strategies which were humiliating and, even now, make me cringe with embarrassment when I recall them. The only way I could manage to walk to the shops was by stopping every so often to sit on the nearest perch. Since there were no seats conveniently placed at the intervals I required, I had to sit on garden walls or steps. Failing that, I sat down on the pavement. In the first days of the illness, when the pain, fever and weakness were acute, I had to ask my parents to come down from Sheffield to look after things while I lay in bed, but as this gave them the chance to spend a bit of time with their nine year old granddaughter, they weren't too put out.

The whole business of this illness was a mystery; this thing which didn't even have a name. No one knew what we were dealing with, nor how long I would take to recover. We all assumed it would be over in a few weeks, but we didn't know. The only direct experience any of us had were childhood illnesses. These were usually over in a week or two, or if they were serious like diphtheria or meningitis, you might die. It didn't enter my head that this was on a different scale altogether; neither getting better nor dying.

Obviously my folks wanted to get back as soon as possible. I was grateful for their help in the emergency, and looked eagerly for the slightest sign of improvement that would allow them to return home, but the fever and pain persisted, and I couldn't manage more than a step or two across the floor. I tried not to let my consternation show.

Dad suggested that we might try an outing in the car. How I longed to get out again! But getting up the stairs from the basement flat was going to be a problem. Maybe today there was just an ounce more strength than there had been yesterday. I was ready to give it a shot. Together, mother and father half carried, half pushed and pulled me, up one step at a time. I felt weak at first, and almost swoony as the car moved off, as if I had never experienced speed and motion before. We drove north to Kenwood House and managed to park just within the grounds.

There was a path leading to the gardens, and it was such a delight to be out in the sunshine among the scents and the flowers, that I was determined to try walking as far as one of the seats. One on either side, they took my weight and almost carried me along the path. This was the furthest I had managed since it all began. Until that day, the effort, even with support, would have immediately brought on an episode of sweating, gripping pains and a crumpling-up of legs. I had feared this when I set out, knowing that if that unbelievable fatigue overtook me while some distance from the car I wouldn't have been able to get back. But now, I sensed something had subtly changed. I felt an uprush of confidence and felt I had taken a real step forward. After resting on the seat for a while, soaking up the colours of the flowers and luxuriating in the warmth of the air, I knew that with their support taking my weight on either side, and proceeding stage by stage with rests every so often, I could make it back.

Oh, this must indeed be the turning point! I was thrilled. The next day came and I felt a degree stronger and even more hopeful. I was able to tell my parents that, quite soon, I would be able to manage on my own. I was sure I was going to recover. At the end of the week I waved them goodbye and turned round to begin my life again. I expected a gradual improvement, but it wasn't going to be that simple. A few steps forward, then a relapse, and more days in bed. Try again! I must do the shopping.

I would set out with my bags and just about get to the end of the road before my strength ran out. Now what? I can't go further, I'm going to fall over. Oh God! I don't want to be lying on the pavement. What will people think? There's nothing to sit on except a wall with sawn off railings. That's going to be rather uncomfortable, but I must sit down. I would sit there until the bits of protruding iron became impossible, and my legs would recover just enough to take me to the next wall. Thus I went about my shopping or taking my two bags of washing to the laundrette.

This was the way for the next two and a half years. The slightest sign of recovery and I would be over the moon, expecting it was coming to an end at last. Then I would start to feel ill again, and what was so depressing was that parts of my body, which hadn't been affected before, were now under attack. New bouts of fever and the biting hot pains began to creep into the tissue of my buttocks and hips, and later into my arms. I had the frightening experience of waking one morning to find that my arms were useless, and cried alone in despair, wondering how I could ever now continue with my sculpture, not to mention all the vital jobs around the house which needed my attention.

Every now and then I visited the doctor again in the mad hope that I would get some help. Yes, he would issue me with the latest antirheumatic drugs and I dutifully took them. They did no good, but gave me a bad case of indigestion. So bad that my intestines, which were very sore and distended as a result of candida, which is one of the symptoms of M.E., became extremely inflamed. It was no use reporting this back to the doctor, as I was to learn that such candour would be met with an exasperated sigh. I read up on the symptoms of the different kinds of rheumatism in the hope that I might come up with ways of overcoming the disease by myself. But although I was to discover that there are many sub-divisions, from osteoarthritis, to the oddly named ankylosis spondylitis, to gout, I couldn't find anything which corresponded to the variety I was experiencing.

I decided to be more clear and specific when I next saw a doctor or consultant. So I reported the fact that I could set out on an errand, walk a few yards with complete ease, with little pain or stiffness in my joints (I could even run a few steps) but thereafter, with each progressive step, my legs would grow heavier, slower and increasingly painful, until after a hundred yards it would feel just as though I had walked thirty miles. If I pushed myself, and tried to carry on by dint of will or mind over body, then, by the time I reached home again, I would be in a state of utter collapse accompanied by the sort of symptoms one only feels with a bad bout of flu. That would result in two or three days of relapse, when I could barely manage to get off the bed, and would have to crawl around on my hands and knees in order to get to the kitchen, where I would prop myself up on a high stool to make us a simple meal. On top of this, even when I didn't push things, there was the constant pain and weakness in my muscles. I tried to point out the painful nodules under my skin, but no one was interested. I told how my eyesight was affected; the blurred vision and red rimmed eyes. Ringing sounds in my ears which I had never experienced before. I could have gone on listing other symptoms, but always at that stage the eyes of the doctor glazed over. He would have stopped listening long ago and would be engaged in swiftly writing out another prescription, this time for tranquillisers or antidepressants.

The fact that the symptoms I was relating didn't accord with a known condition, failed to illicit any kind of honest puzzlement or admission that they just didn't know what to make of it. It seemed to drive them to the only other alternative opinion in their repertoire, namely that I, being a woman, and an abandoned single mother to boot, was naturally an hysteric prone to imaginary aches and pains in order to gain the attention of a male doctor. How many times over the next decade did I hear that phrase 'all in the mind'? It was incomprehensible to me that anyone could deliberately put themselves through such misery, and place such fetters and obstacles on their own life, just to gain the attention of a not very attractive doctor. Or did that phrase mean that one was putting on an act?

I learned to accept the condition, realising that no one was going to help, and work with the good days. Gradually over two years I felt the disease process easing off and giving way to improved health. My hopes began to rise again. I had been so brainwashed by this time, with the constant opinions fed to me by most of the doctors I had seen, to the effect that all I needed to do was pull myself together and get a proper job, that I seriously considered taking a teaching job. I dare say that I would have come to this conclusion around this point without their good advice. My earlier inhibitions, which scared me off from teaching when I first moved to Islington, had been greatly overcome by now. In spite of the handicap of M.E. I had gained more confidence and street-wise experience in the last few years, and besides, my perpetual state of insolvency would have inevitably forced me to get work of some kind very soon.

As my condition improved, my memory of the dramatic details of how it had begun was fading. I began to believe, in the absence of any objective clinical evidence, that all my miserable pain and suffering of the last two years had been – not delusion, I never believed that – but somehow self-created. Wasn't that what psycho-somatic illness meant? My psyche, in its vulnerable, depressed, grieving state, had created, from the landscape of my own body, an outer reality corresponding to the inner scene. Well, this could be possible. The psychologist's casebooks were full of such stories. If this was so in my case then my psyche must be powerful indeed, to have created such a manifestation. Something to be marvelled at! Yet strangely, I thought, no one has pointed this out. All *they* seem to want me to believe is how worthless and ineffectual I am. Yet, however this two and a half years of miserable illness came about, I had survived. I'd struggled on and managed to care for my daughter, keep a five storey house in decoration and repair single-handed, and I'd even done a few sculptures and a folio of drawings and paintings. I will go on to even greater things, I told myself. *And* I will get myself a teaching job.

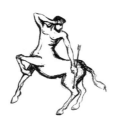

HEALING WATERS

It was in my third year of teaching that I hit on a plan to turn my house into an asset rather than remain stuck with the heavy liability it had become. The glamour of living in London had long since worn thin as far as I was concerned, though not for Sandhya. She was now well into her stride, making new friends and joining in all the activities which Hampstead Comprehensive could offer. She had taken up the cello when she was six, and was now, at the age of thirteen, in the school orchestra. She and her friends were involved in a variety of musical events, from self-composed electronics, and a John Dankworth opera, to classical concerts and even making films. Then there was the school theatre after classes, and of course the usual academic work with O levels in mind.

I had started teaching art in a North London boys comprehensive about the same time that she moved into her secondary school. But after two years with the rough tough boys, I moved to a girls comprehensive in Eastham. I have no regrets about the experiences, the good and the bad, of those teaching years – they helped me to broaden out and develop qualities I probably wouldn't have developed otherwise – but I can't say it was my vocation, and the improvement, which I began to feel three years earlier when I decided to give it a try, had tailed off quite soon after I started teaching.

As anyone in that profession knows, it is exhausting even for the fittest. It was difficult and painful for me to stand up, so the only way I could operate in the classroom was to make sure I had something to sit on at all times, which was somewhat hampering in an art class where you have to be on your feet giving individual attention to the pupils. Then there was the hour and a half journey on the underground to face, morning and evening, battling for a desperately needed seat. I would come home from school at the end of a long, hard day, grab a cup of tea and lie down on the bed, exhausted, and wonder how I was going to find the strength to make a simple meal for the two of us. I couldn't stand up to do the cooking, or the washing-up, but somehow it got done. Then there were the papers to mark and the next day's lessons to prepare, and I would drop into bed feeling sick with tiredness.

This was a dreary existence, and all I had to look forward to was the long summer break. I knew things were becoming serious when the prospect of six weeks holiday, which was regarded by most people as a luxury, just wasn't going to be anywhere near enough for me to regain my strength. The exhaustion was so total that I was sure only six months complete break would do the trick, but that was impossible. What I did plan, however, was a move away from the pollution, noise and aggression of London. If possible, I would try to find a part-time teaching job in some less hectic situation.

What it was that inspired me to move to the Romano-Georgian spa city of Bath, I don't know. There was nothing to draw me to any one particular area in the country. No friends or relations already established in some place which attracted me. I didn't particularly want to return North, even though quite a few of my old friends from the Sheffield days were living in pleasant surroundings, and some comfort, in the Peak District. It was too much of a step backwards for me. But whatever it was that decided me, I suppose must be counted as inspiration. I had just been down for a weekend with an architect friend who had recently taken up a post at Bristol University. He had a house in Bath, and we had driven down from London in his fast, red Saab, and I was returning home by myself on the train. My mind was quite blank with contentment, and was far from any thoughts of house hunting.

We had been at a party the night before, and I'd met some new people with Somerset accents and strange West Country ways, like horse riding and astrology, and we had consumed a fresh salmon, 'poached' in both senses of that word. I was pleasantly relaxed and lazily swaying with the rhythm of the train's movement, when there was a sudden flash of light. Maybe that is too dramatic, but it was as if a window had opened into brilliant daylight. 'Bath is where you must come,' a voice said, and I knew I didn't need to question it. The decision was strangely, and just as mysteriously, confirmed, when, shortly after I had actually bought a house there, and moved in a year or so later, I found myself, one warm afternoon, visiting an outdoor swimming pool. I had never been there before, but as I approached it and walked down a grassy hillside along a zigzag path, stopping half-way to buy an entrance ticket at an old wooden hut, I was aware of a powerful sense of déjà vu. I just knew what was coming next. A semicircular pool of cold water fed by a spring, with ancient semicircular stone arches surrounding the water, came into view through the trees. I had dreamed the whole thing, zigzag path, hut and all, in exact detail some years before.

But at that moment, reclining as I was in the seat of the train taking me back to London, the actuality of selling-up and moving was still some time off. That was a dream of a different kind, and bringing that into reality was not going to be quite so easy. In fact it involved a lot of hard work and quite some stress. It must have taken a good two years. Towards the end of the Sixties, house prices had rocketed upwards, rather like the Eighties boom. On top of that, the street where I had chosen to buy my house, much to my father's disapproval ten years before, was suddenly fashionable and sought after by young up-and-coming T.V. producers and such like. I realised that I had something of value on my hands. I saw my way out. I reckoned I could sell the London house and buy another smaller one in a cheaper part of the country, and still have a fair amount of money left over to invest. This would give me the security of an income to back me while I looked for a part-time job. But as 'oft laid plans' usually do, mine began to 'go agle'. As soon as I put it on the market, property prices took a dive, and the house dropped by about a third in value. Unsold houses were everywhere, and no one wanted it.

Refusing to be daunted, I borrowed some money, contacted Alec, my architect friend, and commissioned him to redesign and extend one of the flats, and convert the rest into self-contained maisonettes. Separate maisonettes would be easier to sell than a five floor house which had been full of tenants, and I might recoup some of the lost value by the time three of them had been sold, as I could ask proportionately more for each. There just wasn't enough money to cover the whole of this ambitious plan, but Alec moved into the spare room, and with the help of a couple of Irish builders, the four of us completed the whole project. It was fortunate that in my last year of teaching at Eastham I had managed to get a part-time post. Three days teaching, two days building, and the weekends somehow-or-other, more often than not, spent in travelling to Bath and tramping the steep streets house-hunting. Needless to say, this was far from the ideal course of treatment for one suffering from M.E., but as I have said, I was following the medical prescription of the time, regarding my aches and pains and fatigue as imaginary and trying to ignore them.

* * *

In August 1975, after some hair-raising financial tightrope walking and some very hard work, Sandhya and I and our little cat packed into a wicker basket, set off on the train to Bath. The new house was a dream come true. We had a sunny garden with wild strawberries, prolific burgeoning roses, and a magnificent view. Everything was propitious and life could start anew. After the exhaustion of the final run-up to selling the three now completed flats and packing up for the move, the peace of the new house in a quiet cul-de-sac was transformational. When the wind was in the right direction, rather than diesel fumes from the Holloway Road in Islington, you could open the door and smell the evocative scent of cows in a meadow, drifting in from the fields behind Beechen Cliff.

I began to recover almost immediately. It was slow, of course, but it was steady. In that first year everything in my life began to take on a new shape and energy. Maybe because those first two summers were exceptionally warm and sunny, the city seemed to vibrate with carnival atmosphere. Every street was alive with excitement and colour. Our arrival coincided with the Bath Festival Fringe and flower power was still holding sway. A mini Woodstock was taking place in the grounds of a derelict church among the gravestones, and people were cooling off by diving into the Avon all along its banks. Even round the weir in the city centre, scantily clad revellers dipped in and out of the water under the frowning brows of the municipal authorities.

At every corner you would bump into someone performing street theatre or juggling. Musicians, mime artists or ballet dancers seemed to take up every available space both indoors and out. Even in the wintertime, when most of the performers had departed, I would walk the streets happy just to drink in the atmosphere of the historic city, feeling the harmony which I sensed issuing from the proportions of the fine Georgian buildings. As well as the vibrant, sensual music of the young, I heard quartets and trios playing Mozart and Bach, Bartok and Stockhausen. It was my city. It was home. I met more people and made more friends in a few months than I ever knew in London. And I met Martin.

We met and fell in love. He was several years younger than me, midway between my daughter and myself. It didn't seem possible. It couldn't work. Yet in all else but age we were matched. We shared the same tastes, loves and passions, and as our relationship lengthened and deepened, we only discovered closer kinship, and possibly more important than that, we knew that our partnership would be one of mutual self understanding, growth and support. These next few years were extraordinary. A sort of renaissance was taking place. However, I couldn't find a teaching job, because at that time teaching posts were being cut back and the crazy official rule was that you could *only* be interviewed for available vacancies if you held a teaching post already. By giving up my job in London I had locked myself out! I decided to fall back on my only skills, which were pottery and sculpture, since without school qualifications I wasn't in a position to apply for other remunerative work. I realised by that time that I wasn't going to make a living through producing huge sculptures, which no one wanted or couldn't afford, so I would try for something less ambitious and make saleable ceramic sculptures. I also did a little private teaching. Then I took up bronze casting and produced three or four small bronzes. After a couple of years I wasn't doing too badly. I had one or two exhibitions where I had sold not only ceramics but the odd few sculptures, and it began to look as though I might make it after all.

The M.E. had not gone away during this time, but I was learning to co-operate with it. I never lost my initial delight in walking round the streets of Bath. Just being there gave me enormous pleasure, and it was as fresh after four years as when I first arrived. Even so, I still had to plan my excursions carefully. Bath was so much more manageable in size and was far more liberal in the provision of public seats, so I could do a hundred yards through town and be fairly sure of a sitting place. It didn't work so well when it was raining, but then I had contingency plans. There would be a café within reach and I could sit at a table and drink coffee. Often these days I would bump into friends and share a table and a chat. Karl Jaeger had opened the Brillig Centre, which was a fabulous meeting place with bouncy, hand-painted armchairs, delicious healthy wholefoods available in the mornings, and avant-garde cinema and concerts in the evenings.

A feeling of gratefulness to the city and to the inspiration that had drawn me to it flooded in when I woke in the mornings. These first four years had brought me renewed health and a wealth of new friends. But I had recently noticed the pain and fatigue occurring more and more often. I put it down to the fact that I was once again preparing for an exhibition and had involved myself with producing a few bronzes to go in it. It wasn't only the casting process that was heavy work, but the fettling, sawing and filing of metal which came after; it took a great deal of energy and muscle power. My absorption with the processes; the excitement of pouring molten metal out of the crucible into the investment and watching the wax disappear, drove out all warning signals from my body of the weights I was lifting and the sheer physical effort I was putting into my work. This time I wasn't ignoring my body's messages on account of some doctor wanting to prove his point about a non-existent disease, I was doing it because I wanted to. My fatigue was irritating and inconvenient for me. It was getting in the way of my own sense of achievement and the fiery, driving enthusiasm of the creative urge.

My energy was leaking away more noticeably each day. I seemed to use up my dwindling quota early in the day, and have to rest for longer periods. As each day wore on, everything became more difficult, until at bedtime, the stairs turned into an insurmountable obstacle. At first I was pulling myself up one step at a time, holding onto the banister rail. I told myself that with a couple of days rest I would feel better, but a few days later I was crawling up the stairs on hands and knees. A trip to the doctor resulted in another version of déjà vu. Here in Bath the doctors were even more scathing about my symptoms, and conservative to a degree. One had the cheek to interrogate me about my lifestyle and ask why on earth I had come to Bath without securing a proper job. 'Trying to live on these bits and pieces of pottery is ridiculous,' he accused me. 'Too many people are playing at being artists. Have you got a husband? No? Tut-tut!' He hands me another prescription for tranquillisers.

Once again branded with the epithet 'psychosomatic', carrying the clear implication that a woman trying to live outside the conventional structures without a husband at her head, was bound to be neurotic. I was beginning to feel a sense of despair, as I was feeling unbelievably ill as the muscular pains and weakness rapidly advanced. But nowhere could I find support. Even Martin, baffled by the lack of medical evidence, tended to disbelieve how dreadful I was feeling and how truly I was being robbed of strength. We were now living together, sharing the house and the household duties. It had been a most harmonious threesome at first, as he and Sandhya had been the greatest of friends. Then Sandhya won a scholarship to a London art college and decided to take a year off before beginning her course. She was travelling by land all the way back from Sri Lanka, where she had stopped to visit her father, and having crossed the sub-continent of India, was now somewhere in Afghanistan, Iran, Turkey or Greece on the last lap home.

Martin and I were both concerned about her long absence with only the occasional letter. This anxiety could have been a factor in my condition, but it certainly didn't account for the whole of the sudden decline. The exhibition was in a few days and I struggled to finish the last few pieces. I put everything I'd got into it in terms of commitment and energy, and was anticipating the satisfaction of a little success and perhaps making a bit of money. This time it was a group show and there would be a party afterwards, so whatever happened, I could look forward to a celebration with fellow artists. Then in a week or two, Martin and I were going on holiday with Lena, to stay in a converted farmhouse in Tuscany, and this was also something I was anticipating with enthusiasm.

Then I fell really sick. It was as though a virus had struck. Fever and pains in my joints and in my kidneys. I was so weak I couldn't get off the couch at all during the day. Martin and I talked it over and decided that we had better call in the doctor, so that if it was something treatable with an antibiotic we could get the treatment underway in time for the three day drive from Bath to Tuscany. It was unthinkable that we would cancel our holiday at the last moment and let Lena down. She was going with us in our car, and it was too late to change plans. The doctor grudgingly visited and prescribed something, but three days later I was worse. Martin wanted to phone Lena and cancel the trip, but I wouldn't let him. 'If I'm going to be ill,' I said, 'I might as well be ill in Italy as in Bath. So let's go.'

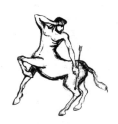

IMMORTAL BIRD AND THE FIREFLIES

In one way or another this decision was to prove fateful. If I hadn't gone, it may be that I would have made a steady recovery in the end, or maybe not. Who knows? But it was during that disastrous/wonderful holiday that Martin and I became more deeply bound in love than ever before. I hadn't anticipated that the journey itself would take such a toll. At lunchtime, somewhere in northern France, we stopped to spend pennies at a motorway rest. I had to have help getting out of the car, and only with the greatest difficulty staggered to the loo. This was to be the last time I was able to use my legs for the next four months. When we finally arrived at the isolated Tuscan farmhouse, in a torrential storm, at dark of night, I couldn't get out of the car and had to be carried into the building and up the staircase where I dropped onto the bed.

All night long I was in a sort of delirium. Flashing lights and streams of vivid colour raced through my head. I told myself it would all come right after I had had a night's rest. But in the morning my legs were burning and when I tried to sit up and put my weight on my feet, struggling to stand up, they folded and crumpled like tissue paper. Martin and Lena fixed me up with a plastic bucket to pee in, but I couldn't squat over it. The only way I could use it was to stretch my weak legs over onto the next bed, and suspend myself over the bucket which was on the floor in the space between. The storms went on for three days and nights, casting an even more gloomy shadow over the proceedings. I was conscious only of my two friends coming and going in the gloom at intervals, as they foraged for food in the village or hunted for the switch for the central heating, but I could barely manage to sit up. I kept dropping into a weird, deep sleep in which I experienced nightmare sensations: I was eternally falling, falling down a shaft, down a well, ice cold, and my heart felt as though it was being peeled of its layers of protective covering until only the most sensitive and vulnerable, pitiful, pulsating core was left at the centre. And all through those dark nights a nightingale kept watch outside my window. She sang her heart-melting melodies, which flooded through my distorted brain, washing out the jagged pieces and calming the zigzag flashing lights, until I was left like a piece of gauze hung out to dry. All my substances seemed dissolved away and my life-force seeped out. I was fading, dying. Would I ever see my home again? There was only this full throated melody outside the window, and lines from Keats Ode to that immortal bird echoing in the darkness, 'Now more than ever seems it rich to die, To cease upon the midnight with no pain, While thou art pouring forth thy soul abroad in such an ecstasy!'

Slowly the storms abated and the fourth morning came in with sunshine. Bluetit fledglings were taking daring little fluttery leaps from one rough jutting-out stone of the barn wall to the next. I could just see them outside the window. That night the nightingale was not so close. She seemed to be singing in a tree a little further off, and she didn't sing as long. Each successive night now she had moved further away, and sung for a shorter time. Her song was as sweet and as mournful, and I wanted to stretch out to her and hold her to me, but it was as if she was weaning me away from her. I was beginning to get stronger. The precious days of our holiday were going by and I hadn't yet been able to join in, but on the fifth day, Martin lifted me up and carried me on his back down the steps to the terrace below my window, which he said was overhung with beautifully scented wisteria. He and Lena had been out and bought wonderful foods which they'd spread on the marble-topped table, and found a lounging chair for me to lie on. At last I was in the warmth of the April air and taking in my surroundings for the first time. We were half way up a mountain and down below in the distance was the blue Mediterranean. All was perfect.

During the second week the nightingale flew away, but her place was taken by fireflies. Martin was bursting to show me these creatures glowing in the dark, and so he and Lena made a carrying chair of their arms and with my arms around their necks we stumbled and lurched across the herby pasture, tripping over the uneven tussocks of reeds. Trying not to make a sound, we made our way down towards the trees, probably looking to anyone observing us in the darkness like some drunken survivors from a wreck. The exertion, even of being carried, drained me until I felt faint, but I had never seen fireflies before, and I wasn't going to miss them. The moon went behind a cloud, and at first it was difficult to make out even the shapes of the trunks and branches, let alone fireflies. Maybe our approach had turned them off, for it seemed we would be disappointed, but soon one luminous greenish light after another switched on, hovering and darting between the leaves. I had expected tiny pinpricks of light, but these were sizeable fluorescent globes, and I held my breath, straining to see more, but I couldn't hold on any longer. It scared me how fast the feelings of illness and fatigue overcame me again even in the midst of a wonderful experience. When at last we got back to the house, Lena and Martin made a wood fire in the big hearth and once more I lay in my lounger feeling the healing energy of the fire soaking into me, as we talked and ate and drank. My spirits were returning though my body was limp and lifeless, and I experienced a great upsurge of life-force, in spite of the fact that my legs were refusing to work. Never before had I felt so positive about the future, as if in defiant contradiction of my physical state.

* * *

The long journey home set me back once more, and my physical condition continued to deteriorate week by week after we returned. We had to resort to calling the doctor again, and even he had to admit now that something was seriously wrong. Through reading articles and hearing items on the BBC, I had diagnosed myself by this time as having M.E., but he would have none of it. I told him that all the symptoms I had been experiencing since the beginning, were the same as the ones described in the articles, but his incomprehensible reply to that was that people always imagine they are suffering from an illness after they have heard a series of symptoms described. I pointed out to him that I had these symptoms consistently for ten years *before* I heard or read the items, but that logic was lost on him. However, he decided to put me in hospital for what was called, 'care and observation,' but that turned out to be yet another deeper shade of nightmare.

The nurses in charge obviously took it from the start that I was putting it all on, as there had been no little bugs helpfully showing up in my blood tests, and they were thoroughly instilled with the idea that M.E. was a fake illness. Some of the junior nurses were more sympathetic, and tended towards a sneaking belief in M.E. They tried to be helpful, but they were going against orders. Those in authority insisted that there was to be no nonsense and no concessions, no help with toilet facilities or with feeding, and I was taken out of bed to sit upright in a chair for the regulation time. I told them that my abdomen and trunk muscles were so weak that I couldn't hold myself upright, but that was ignored. They left me there for an hour and a half, as I slowly slithered down the plastic leather of the chair and slipped to the ground, from which position I could do nothing but lie there on the floor. I was very frightened and alarmed by the unbelievable loss of energy which I was experiencing. Most of the time it was impossible for me to hold any sort of conversation, the effort of forming words and putting them into speech tired me so badly that it was difficult to breathe. Even well-meaning visitors who understood that I couldn't speak, exhausted me by talking *at* me. What they didn't understand was that listening also takes energy.

No one who has not been at that depth of exhaustion can know that even forming a thought takes its quota of energy. Thinking how to lift my arm high enough up to take hold of my fork, and then get it from plate to mouth, had all the complexities of a planned military campaign, when viewed from the slow motion of a completely depleted energy system. Surprisingly enough I was desperately hungry, but the nurses took my food away from me uneaten, because after a few attempts my arms collapsed and I couldn't get my fork to my mouth. All night long, elderly women in the ward talked and snored loudly. They went in and out of the lavatory, banging the door and dazzling me with the lights. The lights and sounds were torturous, son et lumière from the madhouse. I needed sleep like a drowning man needs air, yet the nightly din made me frantic and distraught.

Martin visited me and brought treats, and fed me with strawberries, and real wholesome, health-giving salads, instead of the lettuce leaf and beetroot which the hospital provided as nourishment. I pleaded with him to get me out of the place. Once again I literally thought I was dying. Instead of 'care', the hospital environment was taking away the last threads by which I was clinging to life. And it wasn't just my subjective opinion. I learned later that people who had visited me during that stay, had said to one another that they thought I was dying. It seemed so to me, and I didn't want to die, but if I was going to I would rather do it at home in peace, than in this bedlam.

I was discharged on condition that I would undergo a psychiatric assessment. This turned out to be a complete fiasco. 'We are unable to find any category of mental illness to place this lady in,' was the conclusion. 'She doesn't fit with any known psychiatric condition. We can do nothing for her. She is not depressed, she is not suffering from delusions, in fact, whisper it quietly, she seems pretty normal. It's just that she has this inconveniently undiagnosable er... condition. We pass her back to you.'

I came home. There were a few quiet weeks in the summer. A slight lift in my energy levels, and I managed to get onto my feet for a few short steps. Martin made me a proposition. 'We'll get married if you can make it to the Registry Office and stand up while I put the ring on you.' I was carried up the steps and we were married at nine o'clock on a July morning, in the presence of two witnesses and with Sandhya as 'bridesmaid'.

THE BLACK HOLE AND THE LIGHT

We radiated happiness – remembering the magic we had basked in, which had imbued us with warmth and strength. The sunshine and the wood fires of Tuscany; the positive feelings we had both sensed inside ourselves, that in spite of the calamity that had seemingly overtaken me, there was still a potential and a promise of new life waiting to be unleashed. We must have faith that we could overcome whatever it was that was bent on destroying my life. But there was a sadness too. Why was it that two people who were so clearly meant to meet and to love, had somehow missed each other on the path? Born at the wrong times, and only meeting when it was almost too late? Our fate did seem to have played us strange tricks. We had this opportunity now. This short summer, but we didn't know how short it would be before winter's darkness would come down and test us to the limit.

As the summer waned I became, not only weaker again, but wracked by great storms and convulsions. As though I had been plugged into an electrical socket, shock-waves surged through my nervous system and shook and twisted my body until I was left like a quivering jelly. Pains flooded through me until there was not a cell in my body that escaped the onslaught. I took to my bed hoping against hope that rest would help me, but things only grew worse. Every system was affected. Spasmodic deafness, with high pitched whistles and warbles in my ears, like an old-fashioned radio searching for a channel. Eyes so sensitive that it was painful to focus on anything for more than a few seconds. Breathing, speech, digestion, were all affected, and worst of all I cried now at the least thing. Cried at the waste, the sadness of it all. Why was it all being taken away from me, now, when I had everything to live for?

First my sculpture had been taken away, so I had turned to ceramics, as that might be less physically demanding. When that became too exhausting I tried to draw, but soon that became impossible too. And now I couldn't read, or watch TV, I couldn't talk without exhausting myself. I couldn't write, and could only feed or wash myself with the greatest difficulty. I looked at my weak muscles and felt a pang of alarm. My arm muscles drooped from the bone, slack and without tone, so I tried to do some little exercises in the hope of strengthening them. I grasped my wrists as hard as I could and pushed each of my forearms in opposite directions. I did this two or three times until they dropped down useless to my side, and I lay back exhausted, waiting for my energy to come back. But instead of a gradual return to strength, all the muscles in my body began to twitch, and soon I was shaking and bathed in sweat. Just as though someone had pulled the plug on me, I felt the energy withdraw from my throat, my abdomen, my heart, my brain. I was prostrate, and it was three days before the limited energy I had before I tried to exercise began to return. Obviously I mustn't try this again.

By October I had to have a nurse in to wash me. We were still hoping against hope that the bedrest would effect some healing response, but as we came into November and the symptoms only became more severe, Martin decided to give up his work to look after me. I was in a torment of pain. Sometimes it went on for sixteen hours without let up, and pain-killers had no effect. In desperation I began to take sleeping tablets to knock me out. The few weeks before Christmas I was in such agony that I couldn't even lie flat, since I couldn't find any position which wasn't intolerable. In despair I twisted myself into a half-sitting position, with my knees drawn up and my head turned backwards against the wall. However bizarre this sounds it was the one position which wasn't completely unbearable, and I stayed clamped into that twisted pose all night long outside the bedclothes, wrapped in my dressing gown.

This must have been the nadir. In these few days before the coming of Christmas, I saw blackness oozing up through the floor and forming a pool around the bed. I felt it seeping into me and sickness overwhelmed me. I had deteriorated to the point now where I needed someone to lift me into a sitting position, and to turn me when I lay down. Up until that moment, in spite of the pain and loss of faculties, I had kept hold of hope. Unable to use my hands or talk or listen even, I had one last expression of individuality. I had at least been able to practice meditation. Touching into that higher level of consciousness, I had sometimes been able to rise above the pain for a few brief moments. I had poured out my thoughts and prayers and called positively to the powers of Universal healing and light

But suddenly, I could hope and fight no more. I looked over to where the chest of drawers stood against the wall, knowing that in the top drawer there was a bottle of sleeping tablets. If only I could have crawled or rolled across the carpet to get at them I would have taken the whole bottle. But the pain of movement was too severe, and I was too weak to drop from the bed to the floor, never mind stretch up to pull open the drawer. They were out of reach. So was the window. I couldn't

get to it. I screamed inwardly to God, to the powers of th
have had enough. I want to die.' It was the first and only
said this in my life, and meant it.

That night the pain was bad. As bad as ever it had been, but a
of my bed, about a yard above the floor was an intense, shim. ⸗ring,
oval pattern of blue light two to three feet in length. So rich and deep in
its blueness that there was indigo and violet in its depths. I was astonished, but so weary with the pain I fell asleep.

On Christmas eve, Martin and I slept side by side. Again it had been a
difficult night, and I struggled to turn my painful, dead-weight body
over without waking him. Fitfully dozing, I waited for dawn. I watched
the tiny gap between the curtains where they should have met in the
middle of the window, and I saw the sky outside turn from black to a
deep ultramarine blue, and in the gap was one bright silver star. It
seemed to symbolise the return of Hope.

*　*　*

New Year was exceptionally cold. The temperature dropped to minus
10°C. I thanked heaven that in this cold I didn't have to spend another
night in a twisted and cramped position outside the bedclothes: the pains
had eased off a little and I could lie flat again, though my knees had
stiffened into a bent position and wouldn't straighten out. Ice gripped the
house and the water supply froze up. Every so often I saw the vivid,
beautiful deep blue light within the room. It was as though it was
guarding me. I was sure it wasn't delusion, and I allowed myself to address my thoughts to the presence. I couldn't be certain, of course, but I
felt sure that my questions were being understood and responded to.
Strange synchronistic occurrences began to happen. Visitors arrived
bringing books. Opening one at random, my eyes would fall on a paragraph which gave me clear and immediate answers to urgent questions
which I had posed to the blue light. From one book in particular, Ruth
White's *Gildas Communicates*, I learned of the phenomena of spiritual
guides, and about the power of spiritual healing, and I drank this information in.

Only a short time earlier, I would have regarded behaviour such as this
as gullible and superstitious, but the desperate situation had pushed me
into risking a position which my reason couldn't sustain. Possibly, by
coming to the edge of the precipice I now felt I had nothing to lose. I
allowed myself to experiment more fully with an area of life which I
would never have touched in the ordinary way. I still held on to my rational faculties, so that I shouldn't get carried away by wish-fulfilment

or fantasy, but with time, I began to feel sure that there was a presence from that other world watching over me. I also found I was able to see auras of coloured light around objects in the room.

Simultaneously two other developments occurred. A circle or disk of sky blue light appeared in front of me, shone and disappeared, then shone again. I felt emboldened to address it, when no one was in earshot. 'Are you a guide?' I asked. The light blinked on and off. I blinked my eyes with surprise and asked again. The light twinkled like a star and switched itself on and off several times. 'How can we communicate?' I asked. And immediately I felt an inner response. 'Pick up that book,' it was saying. I did so, and a strange sensation came into my hands as I held it with the page edges facing me. In the tips of my fingers I felt a 'buzzing' sensation and my hand hovered over the tightly closed pages. Then my fingernail sliced cleanly between two pages as though powered by an electrical energy, and opened the page. As I looked down at the page a paragraph lit up. A white light, rectangular in shape and fitting exactly over the printing, illuminated a paragraph of text. And there was a perfect, meaningful reply to my question. I tried this new trick again and again with the same result until I had satisfied my immediate need for response. I experimented with this questioning on several more occasions, as you can imagine, and was amused to see how versatile was my communicator. Sometimes, the heading at the top of the page would be picked out in a rectangle of blue light, while the text was highlighted in white. Sometimes a line or two, and sometimes just a word, would be underlined by a mini fluorescent blue line. And sometimes, just for fun, a tiny ping-pong ball of white light bounced from word to word.

Suddenly I was discovering that the world of the spirit which I had read about before with fascination (but at the same time keeping a healthy hold on my rational scepticism) was proving to be a reality. I marvelled at the phenomena I was witnessing, and simultaneously I was bursting with questions. I went on asking, and usually I was given answers. Sometimes by means of texts in books, sometimes through symbols, or just through amazing synchronicities. The messages rang true and were powerfully meaningful to me. They spoke to an inner place and a deep need. As much as I longed to share my excitement at my discovery with others, particularly Martin, I found no way to convey the truth of what I was experiencing. They, other people, were on the outside, and what was living truth to me, was only as curious or as ridiculous to others as reading about someone else's other-worldly experiences had recently been to me.

The misery of the illness still dragged on. The confinement to my one position and the days and nights of pain continued, but I felt I now had hold of a thread of light which would lead me out of darkness. Spring was ahead, and outside the window I could see blue sky, and the heavy, thick twists of glassy icicles which had formed on the lintels began to drip slow, clear, silvery tears. At first it was only an hour or so at midday before they froze again, but there was a sense of the gradual loosening of winter's grip.

I became quite used to seeing the auras of rainbow colour around the windows and other objects in the room, but was surprised and delighted to observe a new phenomenon: tiny pinpoints of light moving within the room. A few at first. Silver, gold, red, blue. They would appear and disappear. A little cluster in the corner, a few by the vase of flowers. I watched, and they seemed to want to show me how varied they were capable of being. Green in the centre of a flash of gold, or violet within silver. Red with blue, orange, lime green. They came day after day until sometimes there was a throng of dancing points of light. I gave up trying to share this with my visitors; they obviously thought I was going mad!

I didn't feel mad, only entertained and enchanted. But I felt compelled to test my vision out for my own satisfaction. Perhaps my eyesight *was* playing me tricks. After all, my whole nervous system had been shattered and damaged, maybe these were symptoms of physiological disturbance and not fairy-light entertainers. There was a mirror opposite my bed. It was at such an angle that I could see the landing beyond the bedroom door when it was open. The door was to the right of the bed, and when it was open it screened the opening from my sight, but I could see in the mirror anyone about to enter the room. I had watched clusters of these tiny multicoloured visitors many times appearing in different spots in the room, and it was possible that they were figments of disordered vision. But one day, gazing idly into the mirror I saw a cluster of tiny lights in the corridor outside my room, screened from my direct vision by the open door, but plainly reflected in the mirror.

Why I was treated to this entertaining visitation is a mystery. Perhaps they had just come to keep me company through the most difficult days of my life.

MESSAGES FROM THE DEEP

(and the appearance of the Inner Healer)

Three months later, and the new life and new aspiration, which our midsummer marriage had promised, had all too rapidly faded. We never dreamed that, as autumn turned to winter, we would be faced with that king-sized relapse and a slide into nightmare. Nor in our wildest fantasies could we have imagined that we might have such outlandish supernatural experiences to grapple with. As my physical condition had worsened I felt as though I was being sucked down into a black hole, and as I fell and darkness engulfed me, only the grim face of death seemed to await me at the bottom. The end of the struggle, and also the end of all our hopes. But a strange light had pierced the darkness heralded by that Christmas star, and something incredible was breaking through. This powerful, dazzling light had not only appeared, but was attempting to open up communications. However rudimentary, however humorous these techniques for finding ways to convey meaning were at times, they were startlingly and hair-raisingly beyond any normal experience.

At the time, it wasn't possible to see the broader picture. Everything that was happening, from the nightmare of the disease process itself, the boring uselessness of days dragging on and on, to the extraordinary experiences of the Light, were like scattered pieces of a jigsaw, fragments of a mosaic. Some were dark, painful, jagged, pieces, some were dull and blurred. Others surprisingly bright and vivid. Yet taken all together it felt bizarre; a chaos devoid of meaning.

Only now, today, is it possible to recognise that some new design was forming. The disease was breaking me down into fragments, but light was breaking through the cracks. Eyes, which the illness had made too sensitive to watch a television screen or even read, were suddenly able to see levels of reality which they had been blind to before. But that wasn't the only level of consciousness which was breaking through. There was another breakthrough. The wisdom and healing power of my own psyche was also communicating itself to me.

During those long, desperate months of incarceration and pain, unable to change my position in bed, let alone my location within the room, I had only one view – straight ahead. I had a restricted view of the room, but I could see out of the window! I had a panoramic view of Bath and the surrounding green hills in the distance. Apart from that one opening into the world I was trapped inside my distorted body and mind, and each day became a test of survival. Since all the painkillers that had been tried proved ineffective, sleep had been the only escape from intolerable pain. But often that sleep was snatched from the mouth of pain through sheer exhaustion as I became worn out by the relentless torment.

I had sought the benediction of temporary oblivion, but often I would find myself conscious in another world. The world of dreams. At this stage in my life I had some experience of the value and symbolism of dreams, gathered from long years of study and experiential work in psychotherapy. I have described the dark days in London, but out of those dark times had come many rich rewards. I developed a deep interest and passion for the work of C.G. Jung, and had devoted myself to reading his collected works. Also, I had undergone five or six years therapeutic counselling, two of them with an elderly doctor who had himself studied with the great man. He introduced me to painting and keeping a notebook of dreams as a way of working with ones own personal unconscious, and his library was full of rich treasures from the world's mythology which he shared with me.

So I welcomed the series of dreams which now came to me, and I hoped that they would throw some light on my present plight. Although I wasn't able to write anything down, I tried to remember them and unravel their story. I was sure they contained messages and wisdom from my own unconscious which might help me to get at the root cause of the disease and find ways of healing it, if only I could understand them. It was a hard task because I had little energy to decipher their meaning when I woke the next day, as I was being battered into a pathetic shadow of myself by the disease process.

I did begin to extract something however, and piece by piece as I put them together, I thought I could detect definite themes emerging. I kept on meeting a cat. A remarkable cat. Although the creature was in a cat's body and occupied the usual physical situations that a cat normally does. Walked on all fours, ate from a saucer, caught its own food, uttered the same sounds that a cat has always done, yet there was 'a look in its eyes', if I can put it that way, which conveyed the message, 'I am your equal. I know my own knowing, and if I decide so to do, I will let you into my secrets.'

Only it didn't. Not right away, at any rate. At first it went about its business. Did its own things. But we each knew that we were sharing one another's company, and sharing with each other our separate but related worlds. So we just watched one another. Then things took a strange turn. I was following the progress of the cat through some long grass. She was close to the ground, but I could see her pathway as she caused the grasses to wave. She emerged and crossed some open ground, and made towards a damper, reedy patch fringing a pool. Without pausing, she continued her progress and her direction and, just as if the pool hadn't been in her way, plunged in and deliberately swam down to the bottom.

I was astonished. I waited and watched, expecting her to come spluttering up, squealing and hollering, as any normal cat would do who had taken a tumble into a pond. But I waited some time and she did not emerge. Now I felt panic on her behalf. She must have drowned. She'd been under far too long and I couldn't see her in the dark depths of the water. Then up she came with a large fish, the size of a sea bream, in her claws. She was grinning like the proverbial Cheshire feline, as she gleefully deposited the fish on the bank, making it obvious that it was a present for me. Then off she went, well pleased with herself. Needless to say, I puzzled over this for some time.

The Jungian interpretation of this would probably be that the cat, being an animal, represents our instinctual wisdom, as many dream animals do. But being closer to human beings, in that they share our homes and our lives in a way which wilder creatures don't, they symbolise an instinct closer to consciousness. The fish, in contrast, is far removed from us. Water symbolises the Unconscious, as dry land does the more conscious awareness. A fish is a content of the Unconscious.

My dream cat, clearly to me, had a highly developed instinctual wisdom with status equal to but different from human beings. She *knew* in her cat wisdom that I needed to have contact with an instinctual part of myself which lived so deeply beyond my conscious awareness that I didn't even suspect it existed. Human awareness has lost touch with these depths, but the cat wisdom could act as a bridge or messenger which could draw them together again. This she did superbly in her own cat-wise manner.

Another series of dreams brought in a fishy theme. This one stands out in its clarity and its abundant meaning. I am swimming in a strongly flowing stream which takes me into a cool lake. I recognise it as being a place where I swam one hot, dry day when we were travelling through Portugal, because it comes to an abrupt stop just where a new road, running from left to right, has been constructed across it. The foundations put there for the road act as a dam wall just where the lake is deepest. As I react to the sudden halt in the flow of my direction in the water, I am aware of large fish, in the dark, deep water. These are very large, as big as sharks. I get the sense of their aggression, but this doesn't seem to concern me. What does, is the fact that the nearest fish is badly mauled. The water is bloody, and there are pieces of its body floating all around. In particular its tail is almost bitten off and it is in great distress.

When I wake up I am immediately conscious of the pain in my feet. It has been there for some days now and has been frightening. It is hard to describe its intensity, but it was as though my feet had been beaten to a pulp and I couldn't find a position in the bed which was bearable. It was a pain which went on for many weeks and only eased off gradually about a year later. Consequently, the nerves in my feet and legs were severely damaged and my right foot and leg, even now, twelve years later, are still affected. So the dream image reflected, in the aggressive attack on the fish's tail, and on the rest of its body, what was occurring within my system, and perhaps, how it was perceived by the instinctual part of myself. Or indeed, it was a call from my body's instinct to my consciousness for something to be done. Because there was another message in the dream interestingly enough, which I didn't pick up at the time.

The road cuts across the flow of the water and creates a dam. The symbolism of the flow of one's life being abruptly stopped, is clear, but it wasn't until much later that I appreciated the possible meaning of the road going from left to right. In the dream I saw people walking along the road and going off towards the right. The damming of the flow: one phase of life comes to a halt, in order to force one to change direction. The left side of the brain is the more masculine, active, thinking, analytical side; the right hand side is the more feminine, intuitive, feeling and passive/receptive side. And being passive; knowing silence; it is the part of our self which can receive the wisdom of the spirit. Would I ever have found the patience and the discipline in my previous life to devote myself to meditation, or understood the importance of the passive/receptive role in the creative process, if it hadn't been forced upon me?

The next important theme involved several terrifying and chaotic scenes, in which I am driving a car that I can't control, and which takes off at increasing speeds along a rutted pathway and begins to career madly across the countryside (the motor system going berserk). Often I meet boulders in the way, the path cracking up, deep ravines, impossible inclines, torrents of water and sinking mud, but the car races on regardless. It seems to symbolise the breaking up of my nerve pathways and the chaotic and terrifying loss of control which the disease is flinging me into. But it was out of this series of dreams that the beginnings of the healing process came.

A figure began to appear. A doctor. Sometimes a man, sometimes a woman, but I knew it was the same person. He seemed to be watching over the proceedings. Once I met him by the side of a reservoir. I was watching too, in this particular scene. There was a red car parked by the waterside with a young man in the driving seat. There was a sudden, impatient roaring of his engine, as the youth reversed, then accelerated forwards, hitting other cars and clipping the concrete wall of the dam. Then, crashing gears, he backed again, and then shot recklessly forward, shunting other cars out of the way. My heart was pounding as I took in the scene. The mad young devil didn't care a damn for other people's property. Delinquent, hooligan! His selfish, blind behaviour was getting to me, and I felt my anger rising. But the next minute he careered at great speed, breaking through the wall and, flinging the car through the air, he crashed into the deep water and disappeared. Then I noticed the doctor again. He was still standing there, observing the whole scene calmly. My emotional turmoil, my panicky reactions to the death of the young man, were instantly quelled, by the confident, detached, authoritative demeanour of the doctor figure.

I can't explain the dream in terms of logic, but it actually brought about a change in the course of my illness. Very soon afterwards, the doctor appeared again, this time sitting in the passenger seat of the car I was driving, and said to me. 'Well now. Let's take a little run. I think you'll find that things go quite well this time.' I set off and drove down the street, slowly, calmly, and without incident. I felt at last that we were getting somewhere.

As indeed we were. Parallel with the process taking place on the inner levels, I had been receiving help from various sources in the outside world. Martin and I had long sessions when we discussed every possibility we could think of that might help. He had devoted himself to writing letters to scientists, researchers, medics, who believed in M.E., and were going out on a limb in their profession to make known their views. My dear old doctor friend in London, who I had worked with in the past in weekly sessions of psychotherapy, visited me and did all in his power to help by writing personally to eminent figures engaged in research on M.E. He also arranged, at his own expense, a course of megavitamins and other essential elements and minerals which had proved effective in other similar illnesses where the origin was still a mystery. A homeopathic doctor trained in orthodox medicine had begun to visit me, and although after giving the remedies a good trial none of them seemed to make a great deal of difference in the end, their support and concern was invaluable, when faced with the utter hostility of the conservative medical clique here in Bath.

I was also in contact now with an absent healer of much repute, who lived in Derby, and who wrote to me once a month. I had always had at the back of my mind, even in my most sceptical period, the thought that if I was ever to be in the position of being struck down by a severe or incurable disease, I would turn to 'one of those healers', as a last resort. I had moved a long way over the years from that sceptical stance where I regarded healing, in the light of my only experience until then, as a branch of showmanship which worked at the level of suggestibility. But the long empty months in which I had lain immobilised, had provided me with the opportunity to do some thinking and some meditating. It had occurred to me that if, as those scientifically minded medical experts believed when they talk of a psychosomatic illness, a person can make themselves sick in the most convincing manner by creating clearly observable effects in the physical body, such as asthma and eczema or heart disease, then the same power could be tapped to bring about a healing effect in the body. If the psyche can affect the soma (the body) in a negative way, which is what is usually meant by the term psychosomatic, then it can affect it positively as well. If elements in our personal psyche can *create* disease in our body, then surely, it follows, that there are forces within us that have the power not only to restore the state that was, but bring about an even greater degree of health. (Although, I have never heard a professional medical expert make this point.) If these unseen powers were at work within our personal psyche, then that part of our consciousness, joined with our conscious intent, could receive a boost of healing energy from the Universal Source. I was quite willing to believe that certain people had the gift to channel that healing power.

Several friends had offered to put me in touch with various healers, and I was considering giving it a try. One friend told me of a Distant Healer who lived in the Midlands who had a great reputation and many successful cases. Distant Healing was as effective as the 'hands on' variety, I was told, so I decided to go ahead. We contacted him and he very kindly agreed to take me on. He said he would write to me about once a month, and Martin was to send him periodic reports since I was incapable of writing myself. And so my experience of healing began.

Nothing the least bit dramatic happened, I have to admit, but there was a slow, gradual improvement. As I have said, the support of all those good and caring people was invaluable, and maybe the combination of all the various approaches was having an effect. The homeopath gave me great encouragement and devised, with Martin, some gentle passive exercises. I had become terrified of attempting exercise after the experience I had had before, when it had sent me into a severe relapse, but at the same time I knew I was in a cleft stick. Without any exercise at all my muscles would deteriorate even further. So we began very gingerly, and with enormous patience, to build up my strength a fraction at a time. By the end of the summer, one year exactly since the devastation began, the two of them lifted me out of bed and held me in an upright position. It was wonderful, even though they were taking all my weight and there was no question of me standing myself. Supported in this position my toes touched the floor but my heels remained an inch or so above the ground. This was because the tendons at the back of my legs had shrunk from lying all those months in bed with toes outstretched. Any long-term bed-ridden person should have had a block to rest their feet against, so that the feet would be positioned with the toes pointing upwards. We discovered this later from a book Martin had bought on taking care of long-term patients. The problem of contractures was pointed out as an elementary mistake to avoid, but our G.P. had never thought to mention it! We were very concerned to discover, after attaining this vertical position for the first time in a year, that I had developed contractures so badly that even my hip joints couldn't be straightened out.

One step forward only to discover another setback, but I had to take it a day at a time. Six months before, I could not have been lifted into that position, I would have suffered the tortures of hell, and I think I would have died. Things *were* improving and hope *was* returning, and I was working very hard to maintain it. Two ladies were visiting me every week to give me healing now, and I began to noticed the positive effect of these sessions. My parents sent some money, and Martin bought a reclining chair with it, which he put beside the window with the hope that it might tempt me to move from the bed. This irrational terror of moving still clung to me. In the months when the illness was at its worst and I seemed in a constant state of delirium, his attempts to move me had thrown me into terror and panic. The insecurity of changing my position brought on nightmares and delusions, as if by moving the bed a few feet, or changing its angle, I had moved into another reality – like Alice stepping through the looking glass. A shift in position stirred some chemical reaction in my brain, and I seemed to step through a hole in the floor of my reality, and all manner of hallucinations would invade me. I knew it was the effect of the disease process, but it overwhelmed me.

But now, with the appearance of the calm and confident healer figure on the inner level, and my own grasp of the steering wheel of my own vehicle, I felt I could begin to trust the old outer realities once again. So I allowed Martin to lift me out of bed and into the chair. There were a few initial wobbles, but the joy of being closer to the garden and the outside view was indescribable, and I clung to the windowsill until the wobbles passed. Soon, we were attempting an even more daring exploit.

Martin managed to carry me downstairs to the bathroom, and we rejoiced in this incredible event: expensive soap, and my hair washed in shampoo for the first time in many months, was luxury beyond belief. Then, as the weeks went by and the improvement continued, my healer in Derby suggested that I should go out in the car for a little ride and get some fresh air. Somehow Martin managed to carry and wheel me, from my bed and into the front seat of the car. Life seemed to be returning in abundance, and by October, when we were offered a little flat by the sea for a week, we thought we should attempt it. It was an hour and a half drive. We knew it would throw my system into some chaos and be quite unpleasant, but with luck, it might only take a day to recover, and the reward would be worth the risk. I did need to spend a day in bed after the drive, but after that we ventured out, with the smell of the sea in our nostrils, on to the promenade. I drank in the space, the expanse of sky and sea, with a feeling of gratefulness for being alive and for just being there with Martin beside me, when, six months before, I had not thought I would survive. And when Martin tucked me up in rugs in the wheelchair and capered at speed across the wet sands, with the October wind streaming out our hair and flapping the rugs, we felt elated and transported with hope for the future.

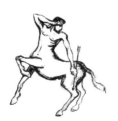

RELAPSE AND BREAKTHROUGH

November came and things stood still. The family were coming to stay at Christmas and everyone was looking forward to a modest cele-bration. My parents had been relieved and delighted at the news Martin had relayed to them over the summer about the signs of recovery. But in the run up to Christmas and the start of the colder weather I began losing ground. Things were not going well, and all of a sudden my muscles began to falter. The twitching returned, the fever, the pains intensified – the lot. Fear began to engulf me once again. I felt that the messages from my unconscious must have let me down. Really, we had tried everything now. There was nowhere left to go, and I clung desperately to the ragged shreds of hope, the sureness I had felt so deeply, that the path to recovery had actually begun. I felt then, at that lowest point of the year, coinciding with the winter solstice, that I couldn't face a shattering re-lapse and having to build up the constructs of mind, body and spirit once again out of nothing. But then came the most significant dream of all.

I found myself walking down the Islington street where I once lived – a terrace of houses running alongside the Regent's Canal. I noticed a young cat who appeared to be in quite a bad state. Her fur was missing in places, and the skin beneath it was bloody. Whether she had been in a fight, or if these wounds were the result of a disease, I couldn't tell. But as I came closer, I was shocked at the pitiful state she seemed to be in. Limbs half severed, tail bitten almost through, eyes damaged, ears eaten away. It was a heart-rending sight and I wanted to do something to help her.

I called to her and communicated my concern, and that I wanted to help. I put my hand out to touch her. My instinct was to pick her up, take her home and look after her, but she was so damaged that it would be difficult. Things were so bad with her that I knew I wouldn't be able to save her myself, but I felt sure there was a vet living close by. But how could I lift her without hurting her even more? I had to try. As I stretched out my hands to her she moved out of reach. I knew that she was aware of my intention to help her, and I was surprised that she even had the strength to move, but I persisted and tried again: she moved again. We continued like this for some time, and I began to see that, in spite of her terrible pain and the seeming impossibility of her being able to move on those severed limbs, she *was* moving in a purposeful way. She seemed to be leading *me* along the path, stopping every now and then to turn round and look at me to see that I was still following.

She was leading me, I realised, to the vet's door. It seemed that *she* knew where it was and realised herself that she needed to get his help. And sure enough she found the way. As we got to the door we saw that the surgery was on the higher floor and that we would have to climb a flight of stairs (symbolic of a shift in levels) so she let me pick her up. By this time I was in a state of near panic, for I wasn't sure if she was going to survive: she seemed so lifeless. I was almost in tears when we were admitted into the vet's surgery and I held out the poor cat for him to see.

He calmed me down right away by his manner, and told me that he would operate at once and was sure that he could save her life. Feeling this surge of confidence in him, I let myself relax and looked around. The first thing I noticed, for I hadn't had chance to notice anything until then, was that it was a very unusual surgery indeed. There was an operating table with sterile sheets, bandages, and all the usual drugs and equipment, but right alongside the sterile table was a tank of murky water with bits of clay and plaster floating about in it. It was a plaster-casting tank from a sculptor's studio. A very familiar piece of equipment to me. We had one just like that in the casting room at the Royal College big enough to take life-sized plaster casts.

For those unfamiliar with it, I will describe the process of casting from clay into another more permanent material such as *ciment fondu* or cold-cast bronze. Suppose that you are working on a life-sized figure. After your original model (which is sculpted in clay) is completed, you proceed to the next stage, which involves sectioning it into removable pieces by using shims of thin brass. Then the clay is covered, section by section, with several coats of wet plaster until a substantial thickness is arrived at. After sufficient time for hardening the whole thing is wheeled by one or two strong assistants into the casting room and lowered into the tank. By that time of course it is extremely heavy. Next, a good soaking, maybe twenty-four hours or so, after which the sections are carefully prised apart and the plaster cast is removed from the original clay. Finally, after drying out and reassembling, these pieces form a hollow mould, which is then ready for the new material to be poured or laid in.

All of this was heavy work, as you can imagine, but it had been one of the operations which I enjoyed to the full in the days of my apprenticeship. It was always wonderful when, after working away on your clay model, sometimes for many months if it was a large and complex piece, wrestling with the creative process – getting blocked – unable to go further with your work, you came eventually to the point where you felt it was finished. Or as near as it would ever be. After all those feelings of frustration, despairing at times that you would never crack it, you would get away from your intransigent lump of clay for a while and have some fun. Sharing your problems with friends, you'd have a few laughs, a few drinks in the pub or a meal in a restaurant, then the 'block' would move. You'd find new inspiration and impetus, come back to your work, and eventually it would all seem to drop into place and you would finish.

The next stage, the heavy work of the casting process, was a bonus. When the new material was set inside the plaster you would get to work removing the mould with hammer and chisel. Transformed into an altogether different material, which might be a shining, golden bronze, your work would appear beneath the chisel, as bit by bit the plaster chipped off.

Returning now to the dream where two impossibly incompatible scenarios stand side by side – the clean, hygienic operating table and its shiningly sterile scalpels, and the murky, fetid water of the casting tank. In real life you would have balked at placing your trust in such a setup, yet in the dream it felt right. Unusual, but right. I had a perfect trust in this vet, who, by the way, was none other than the doctor I had seen before, but this time in another variant of his/her manifestation.

He gestured to me to place the poor body of the little cat on the operating table and I did so feeling quite confident, in spite of the fact that she was showing little sign of life at that instant. I knew in my heart that he would heal her. But at this point I began to be aware of a significant change: a feeling, a sense of new energy. It was momentous. Something extraordinary was about to happen and I was in breathless anticipation. Was I perhaps about to witness some miracle?

But he paused, scalpel in hand, and turned and spoke to me. 'Would you like to help me with this operation?' he asked, and his words awakened what must have been an unconscious need. I knew, in that instant, that more than anything on earth I wanted to be invited to *co*-operate. I needed to be promoted to that position, on an equal level with him, and I knew I could take up the challenge. But at the same time I was trembling with the sense of honour and responsibility which had been invested in me. I told him that in order to be worthy of that honour and the confidence he had placed in me, I would need to participate in some ritual or initiation ceremony. A kind of certification of my status. 'What do I need to do?' I asked.

'That you must decide for yourself,' he said.

'But,' I objected, 'I really don't know. Can't you tell me please.'

'No. But you will soon know for yourself,' he replied.

And then I *did* know. I knew I must put my right hand, the hand which I would use for carrying out the operation, into the murky but sacred water of the tank, and that would be an act of purification which would confer on me the ability to heal. There the dream faded, but when I awoke, I still knew that something had irrevocably changed in my life.

* * *

But outwardly nothing had changed. Every day continued the same. The same misery, the same pain, the same uselessness. Yet I strongly believed there *had* been a change. A week or two later I began to get severe pains in my right hand. It had been weak and useless for a long time, but now, with the pain, it began to seize up. All the joints in my fingers stiffened and the tendons tightened so that I could no longer bend my fingers. On one of his rare visits, I showed my hand to my G.P. and told him that I couldn't bend my fingers. I could see that he didn't believe me even then, and when he took hold of my hand and tried to bend the fingers himself, I was sure that he was hoping to prove a point. 'Look, they will bend quite well you see,' he would have said, 'if only you try hard enough.'

But although he tried with all his might, the knuckles stayed firmly locked, and it was obvious there was a solid encrustation of crystalline deposit cementing the joints together. He gave up and muttered something inaudible and left. It had been pretty painful to have him attempt to bend them, but not much more than the pain I was in anyway. As time went by, however, and the joints stayed locked, I did begin to doubt my dream somewhat. The other hand was also beginning to be affected, though in a different way. The flesh became flaccid and numb, as if it was dying. It felt to the touch just like the cold, unresilient flesh of a cod fish that had lain on a slab too long. This gave me some cause for concern. Yet I managed to cling on to my faith in my inner healer, in spite of creeping doubts which the relapse had caused once again.

Then, something quite extraordinary happened. There was an unexpected phone call from the healer in Derby. Martin had sent the occasional reports for me, but recently the progress had been slight, and with the relapse we probably felt rather ambivalent about continuing to write. Maybe my scepticism about spiritual healing was getting the upper hand again. I was lying in bed as usual, in pain and rather miserable. It seemed my life, such as it was, was fated to be immobilised and confined to the four walls after all. The only change now was that Martin had made a bed for me in the ground floor room on a divan, and sometimes I could sit up for a while and be wheeled to and fro in a wheelchair around the room. The telephone was in the kitchen on the floor below, and I heard it faintly ringing and Martin answering it. A few moments later he came up to tell me that it had been our healer in Derby.

The message which Martin relayed to me was: 'I was concerned at not having heard from you for some time. So I was tuning in to your wife prior to sending her some healing, and was surprised to pick up, tele-pathically, a strong message which said that she is in great need at this moment and that I should contact her, as well as send out some powerful healing. Tell her to prepare herself to receive the healing at five o'clock, by lying peaceful and still in a darkened room for about twenty minutes. Then do let me know if she notices anything unusual afterwards.'

So promptly at five, after Martin had drawn the curtains, I relaxed on my back with my arms at my side. I lay there for the twenty minutes, but, anticipating a lessening of pain, all I felt was a slight tingling in my right hand. Martin duly reported that back, but our Healer seemed a little disappointed as he had 'belted out a lot of healing energy', as he put it. 'Never mind,' he said, 'just let me know if anything more happens.' I think by this time, I wasn't expecting anything more. But an hour later the tingling was stronger, and it continued getting more pronounced all evening. When I woke in the night it was still there and was spreading up my arm. The next morning it was so strong that the muscles began to twitch and, in the fingers of my right hand I felt such strong sensations that the hand seemed to be lifting itself off the mattress. The fingers were twitching and itching and showing signs of a minute flexing and contracting movement which I couldn't control.

This continued and intensified as the day went on. By this time I was so astonished that I deliberately checked myself to see if I was causing the movements. But it was involuntary, like when a large muscle twitches and you can't control it. I allowed my arms to lie completely limp and relaxed by my side, and observed that the right arm was lifting itself off the mattress and coming back down again to rest, and the fingers were bending ever so slightly – painfully – and ever so creakingly, not so much of their own accord, but as if another hand, a very much more powerful hand, was inside my own.

This incredible sensation and movement continued. It would rest for a while and the arm would lay limp. Then the sensations would begin in the nerves, and the palm of my hand would contract from the flat, re-laxed position and arch into a curve, so that the palm was hollow, and then it would straighten out again. Then, as if a deliberately planned set of exercises was being performed, first one tightly locked finger, then the next, would be bent by an inside force. One joint at a time was flexed as far as it was possible, then extended, and the next knuckle would take its turn. I endured the pain, as I watched fascinated and mystified. By the end of the week three fingers had got their flexibility back, so that it was possible to bend them with the other hand. One finger joint remained obstinately locked still, and I didn't have quite enough strength to bend my fingers unaided by my other hand.

I tried to tell Martin what I was experiencing, but his expression communicated his confusion and disbelief more than his words. 'You're trying to tell me your hand is moving all by itself? Oh Esmé!' He said. There was more to come, however. This incredible thing was happening to my right hand, but elsewhere I was in distress and a great deal of pain. I was confined to bed again and barely able to move and sometimes the pains were intolerable. There was a particularly vicious pain in my chest, just above my heart, and I think I was in tears sending up prayers and pleas for someone up there to help me. Martin brought me a cup of tea and helped me to sit up to sip it, then he went away again. I was propped up on the pillows, but crumpled up sobbing and hugging my chest. I'd forgotten my arms for one moment, and I let the right one drop down and rest on the mattress. The fact that it was tingling again seemed of little importance now.

Then I felt a new sensation, as though something, a current of energy, was flowing through my hand. The tingling grew stronger, and the sensation of my hand and arm beginning to lift upwards finally drew my attention. I can only say I watched in amazement as my hand rose up in front of me as light as a feather, and the fingers loosely pointing towards my body began to give out a stream of energy directed at my chest. I saw a stream of vivid translucent colour emanating from my fingers. This poured out for several minutes and was followed by a sensation in the crown of my head. A great light and force came down through the top of my skull, and like the force which took over my hands, it began to bend my spine, pressing my head hard down on my chest. Then it relaxed and let go. Then it began again. Each time it relaxed there was an expellation of energy from the place in my chest where the pain was at its greatest. And each time it was expelled – and it came out as a spurt of energy right through the flesh and bones – the pain receded until it had gone altogether.

Now things really began to happen. In the next few weeks this extraordinary force went to work on me. I was taken in hand and put through a course of exercises designed to get my poor body back into some sort of shape again. My hand would rise up weightlessly and start to emanate healing energy, directing it to different parts of my body. I soon noticed that it would stop and give out an extra powerful jet of light at certain places all down the centre of my body. I recognised that these places coincided with chakra points which I had seen on figures illustrating Hindu yoga manuals. This had all been a bit esoteric for me in the past, and I hadn't taken much notice of their significance, but it was as though the penny had dropped suddenly, and I realised that they must be subtle centres for receiving spiritual energy.

I became aware now of a chakra at the top of my head, the Crown Chakra, as I was to learn later. It would open up and a powerful force would flow in, and I knew it was time for some vigorous exercises. The force would work rhythmically downwards through my neck and chest, bending my spine forwards, flexing and releasing it. It would then push me forward at the lumbar region forcing the top half of my body to bend until my head was touching my feet. It took a few days before this could be done completely, but when the time seemed right, the bones in my pelvis seemed to dissolve and slide with ease into a doubled over position, such as I had never been able to achieve even when I was much younger and at my fittest. Although it was comfortable if I went with the force which had entered me, if I tried to sit upright again or were to try to resist, I found that I was held in a vice like grip and could not move from the position which I had been put into, until I was suddenly released. Then I could sit up easily.

In order to cooperate, and because I wanted to do everything I could to strengthen myself and make as much of a recovery as possible, I sat on the edge of the bed with my feet on the floor several times a day. My muscles were so weak that a sitting position was exhausting, but I positioned some pillows to give me support. In spite of all I had recently experienced, the shortening of the tendons at the back of my legs caused me some dismay. Even if the amazing healing power could help me to get my muscles strong enough to begin the task of learning to walk again, wasn't I going to be permanently crippled? Once contractures have set in, so our book informed us, it would be impossible to correct. I sat there contemplating this new obstacle.

I was taken by surprise. The force got to work again. As I was sitting there with my hands weakly resting on my knees, and my feet, or as much of them as would touch, upon the floor, the strange sensations began again. It was always a great irresistible power which seemed to take over and come down through the top of my head. This time I felt its strength enter my arms and begin pressing heavily on my knees, forcing the heels downwards. Just as with the fingers, the pain was excruciating as the tendons were stretched, but I could not cause the power to desist.

It was immense. Yet if I asked it as a prayer, 'Please, whoever you are, I don't want this,' it would stop immediately and it would be as if nothing had taken place. I felt assured that it wasn't my will that was being taken over, and that however immense the power, it was only operating by my consent.

Getting the Achilles tendons back into shape took weeks of persistence, as it was a bigger undertaking than the fingers had been. But improvements did come gradually, and as if it had been planned, an NHS physiotherapist contacted us and arrived with a walking frame just at the right moment for me to begin the enormous task of attempting to get on my feet and take my first step.

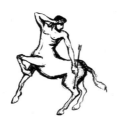

I AM THE HEALER OF MY LIFE

To detail every step along the path towards recovery from this point, would be tedious. It took a great deal of time and patience and a lot of hard work. I could give details of how the powerful healing energy set about detoxifying my body, but that was not a pleasant experience. It was like being put through a mangle. Every cell of my body it seemed was saturated with unpleasant substances which had to be thrown out, but the power flowing through and moving my hands began massaging every inch of every muscle in my body. There was an accumulation of crystals in many places, especially around bony protuberances. Surprisingly, even the bridge of my nose and inside my mouth received determined attention. The deep fingertip pressure drove out the pollution and brought it up to the surface, where it was presumably carried away by fluid systems and eliminated. This made me alternately burn and shiver and feel extremely nauseous to the point where my faith began to waver; I felt so sick and poisoned. But I was shown in an amazing light display how the healing system was working for me. The bedpan, which was constantly (and embarrassingly) within reach, was pointed out to me. This, I was shown, was the most important piece of equipment in this stage of the proceedings. 'We are working extremely hard to rid you of this poison and here is where the pollution is ending up,' I was told firmly. I asked this several times, as usual, not trusting that I had received the message correctly. 'Yes, you have heard correctly', the messenger said, and to emphasise the point the interior of the white plastic bedpan lit up with a beautiful, vivid violet light. Just to make it even plainer it lit up and switched on and off six times.

This is just one incident out of many that took place on the long path to recovery. How I was literally 'moved' by this amazing power off the bed and onto the ground, and then lying and sitting on the floor, was put through a series of yoga-like exercises, is another story. It became apparent that the M.E. condition itself, and then the immense input of light/energy, had left me 'ungrounded'. A whole series of exercises were devised by the 'other world' healers supported by their communication. How I was supported and guided in my attempts to learn to walk again (holding on to the walking frame at first) by asking the advice of my discarnate friend on how far I could go at one session without overdoing it, and bringing on another of those famous relapses, is yet another story. My 'Blue Star' seemed to be joined by a team of healers and helpers on the 'other side' on a 24 hour basis. Always someone there when needed.

The communication and support system from the other world was now being ever more closely and meaningfully integrated with the unfolding of my own inner knowledge. Though progress had to be worked at, and was frustratingly slow on the physical level, there was for the first time a sense of flowing with 'my truth'. I was now sure that real healing was underway. A new sense of confidence in my own process had come into being and at the same time I felt guided and supported by spiritual presences who had my well-being at heart. I began to keep a notebook to record my questions and ponderings and the replies I received from 'Blue Star'. These early attempts at communication were often rudimentary, as sometimes I was lucky enough to 'hear' a few words clearly inside my head, but more often ideas would be conveyed by means of symbols or pictures. I would 'see', rather like a vision, a very quick but vividly clear image whose meaning would be instantaneous. Often this insight would be so fast but fleeting, that I would doubt my instant understanding. But I learned to trust them more and more when my second and third thoughts, which came from my slower, logical thinking processes, proved wide of the mark time and again, and the first impressions proved right. It was a process of trial and error, and I was learning to build my own understanding of this new reality out of each brick of new experience, just as a child learns to understand the material world it finds itself in.

With no previous knowledge to guide me, I had to learn to pick my way through a tangle of possible sources of message. Was I being deluded? If not, then when were the voices coming from my own mind, and when from a true source outside and beyond myself? Could it be possible that I was occasionally picking up voices of mischievous or even malicious entities? It was a minefield. Gradually though, I did learn to discern the resonance of the personality and 'voice' of my 'Blue Star': the one I came to call, Astrazzurra. Over time, and by keeping a notebook of all our conversations, there began to be a recognisable and consistent quality.

For most of the year which followed the breakthrough of healing and the appearance of light, I was still having to spend the best part of my time lying on the bed in the downstairs room, sleeping for long periods and exercising a little at a time. I still needed daylong care, and we thought that I would make much quicker progress if Martin and I continued to

215

work at it together in a positive way, rather than being alone in the house hour after hour, relying on a rather sketchy service of 'meals on wheels', and sparse visits from health visitors and home helps. So Martin postponed his ambitions to establish himself in landscape design and construction for a while longer, and we continued to exist on 'Invalid Care Allowance' and my sickness benefits. He was making good use of his time at this period, when not actually engaged in the immensely beneficial therapeutic support he was giving to me, redesigning and reconstructing our garden. One day he came in from building some steps holding his arm, which was giving him pain. It was an old injury which had never healed properly. It flared up whenever he put too much strain on it. The accident happened when he was about eighteen, and at that time he had been mad about motorbikes. He had been tinkering about with his current model, trying to loosen a tight bolt. He strained with all his might, putting his weight behind the screwdriver, when it slipped and went right through the palm of his hand and out through the wrist.

This accident put him in hospital for some time, and when he was discharged, there was still some matter embedded inside a tendon, and the tissue had grown around it leaving a wound which hadn't healed in spite of the antibiotics he had been given. It ached and remained a permanent weakness. As he sat on the stool beside my bed holding his aching arm, I had a sudden thought. Could I try giving healing to him? The possibility of me being able to channel that healing energy, which had flowed so abundantly to me, to another person, had never occurred to me before. I had talked often about my experiences to Martin, but he had remained sceptical. He was having intellectual difficulty in accepting something of which he could have no personal experience.

Yet he had witnessed such positive improvement taking place in me that he was impressed enough to accept that something outside the ordinary was happening. So I tentatively asked him if he would like me to try. His response was ambivalent, but he agreed. 'I know that you believe you are seeing coloured lights and that they are healing you, but I cannot believe something I can't test and see for myself. But you might as well try it on me if you want to,' was the gist of his reply.

It put me on the spot. I didn't know at that stage if it was possible to transmit this healing power that I was experiencing to others. If I failed then his scepticism would be justified, and although *I* wouldn't begin to doubt what I had experienced, I might feel more freakish and isolated if this knowledge couldn't be shared, particularly with people nearest and dearest to me. So it was with some trepidation that I asked him to move closer, sit on the floor and rest his back on the side of the bed. I invoked my healers, asking them to work through me and give healing to Martin if that was possible. Almost immediately, I felt that energy flow through me and my hands begin to move as if directed by an outside force. They moved in a most precise way as though seeing inside his body. I observed the operation. The force carried my hands across his body and paused over his head, neck, spine, elbow and at a place an inch or so beyond his fingertips, to give out a strong jet of energy. I could not have thought this up for myself.

I noticed too, that within half a minute of the healing flow beginning, Martin had fallen into a peaceful sleep. (I now know from experience that the effect of the healing energy very often acts upon the system, bringing about a deep level of relaxation, a vital ingredient of the healing process.) Whilst he slept, the flow continued for twenty or thirty minutes, then came to a gentle stop. It felt extraordinary. I softly touched him and spoke, telling him that it was completed, and he awoke. 'How do you feel?' I asked. 'Oh! I've had a really nice sleep,' he said. 'But were you aware of anything happening? The healing?' I asked. Hardly able to contain my curiosity. 'Oh! I had forgotten that,' was his only comment.

I was left in suspense, but hardly daring to persist with my need to know. Something *must* have happened. It had been such a wonderful and surprising experience. But I had to let it go. I must not get hung up on expecting immediate results. But the next morning I just had to ask again. This time he told me that his arm had been particularly painful that night after the healing. It had felt hot and aching. 'Oh dear!' I thought. 'What has gone wrong? That wasn't at all successful.' But that evening when I inquired again, he said that in spite of another day's work, it had only given a few slight pangs. The next day the report was that it had been almost without trouble. From that day onwards, there has been no further problem in spite of years of similar hard work.

This experience led me to try this new-found power on others, and I found that my experiences were being confirmed over and over again. One of my regular visitors one day asked me to try giving him healing for a headache. He sat down on the floor by my bed and I 'tuned in' to the healing flow. My hands once again began to move of their own accord, travelling over his upper body about an inch from his skin. They seemed to be sensing, looking for places where the healing energy could be imparted to give the maximum effect. Again, my mind watched without interjecting its own ideas or interfering with the process. I was observing, in a completely detached way, how the energy flowing from my hands seemed to be imparted to the aura and to chakra points. Then, I was taken by surprise when I felt a change of frequency. My fingers made contact with my friend's face and began probing gently around his upper jaw. They found a spot and started to target a much stronger jet of energy directly at it. This carried on for a few minutes and then it was all done.

I was completely puzzled, but before I had time to say anything, my friend spoke. He thanked me for relieving his headache, but what was more amazing, he said, was that I had also found the exact place where his tooth had been giving him hell all morning. He hadn't told me about this and I had no idea beforehand.

From here on my recovery was slow but sure. The mode of healing too was changing, though so slowly I didn't realise it at the time. The intensity of the energy being poured into me day and night lessened and the phenomena of other-worldly interventions, that had been so amazing at first when I had been bodily moved from within, shaded off gradually. Receiving healing and learning to give healing now went hand in hand, and I was able to give healing more often and more strongly as my need to receive diminished. I was gradually becoming aware, not only of the need to share this power with others, but of the responsibility it would place on me to develop a greater understanding of the whole field of spiritual healing. These first experiences of channelling healing, gratifying as they were in the almost supernatural results they achieved, only served to reveal to me what was possible. Even a miracle healing, astonishing as it may be, only demonstrates in a very intensely speeded up and magnified way, the powers of recovery inherent in the physical body. It doesn't give us insights into why disease comes about in the first place. If the person who received the miracle hasn't arrived at that place of conscious balance where disease is no longer possible for them, they could well fall foul of the syndromes which cause illness to manifest again. Fear, denial, suppression, stress or guilt all have the power to bring about dysfunction and ill health. Realising unconditional love allows healing.

I had been given a powerful demonstration of what the brilliant spiritual energy was capable of, and that gave me courage and confidence to go on with my personal healing process and spiritual growth, yet I knew there would still be much to learn. It took time however, before I began to understand the many layers and depths involved in true healing. In the space of a handful of years I would find myself with a number of clients coming to me for healing, and I would be holding twice weekly healing and meditation groups in my house.

Although I was still restricted by fatigue and weakness in the first year or two, I managed to pace myself and use the times when my energy was stronger to begin moving back into life's current. I wasn't altogether free of the fear of triggering a relapse either. Former experiences must have etched themselves deeply into my mind/body system. But now, I had a growing confidence in my spiritual support system. I was being guided at each stage; taught how far I could go and when I needed to slow down. I could call upon my Inner Healer and on the Universal healing energy which was channelled to me, and I could actually see the wonderful colours streaming through. My trust was being built step by step. What if I had lost my ability, for the present, to draw and sculpt? With this spectrum of living colour flowing from my fingertips and en-circling the room, I felt a new mode of creative expression manifesting itself. New possibilities were opening out which I could never have imagined possible.

Although the pleasure of venturing forth, making contacts and meet-ing new people was still restricted, synchronistic events brought once again the right people at the right time, and previously unimaginable possibilities fell smoothly into place. My house became a centre for healing, and later for the establishment of workshops. We held vigils for peace at a time of great instability in world events, and group medita-tions when the light and healing energy that was generated was tangibly present. We formed energy links with other Light Workers in other places with the intent of maximising the gentle power of healing for the world. And the Berlin wall came tumbling down and Nelson Mandela walked free.

* * *

Today my health has returned in great measure and personal horizons have opened out. I have become a voyager both of inner worlds and outer, travelling deep in rural France and embracing the mysteries of Aegean islands. Voyages which have enriched my soul and deepened my understanding. Martin's support has continued, and our relationship has developed into a truly spiritual partnership, as his own inner journeyings yield fruit. I am walking further and more strongly as each day passes, but I am walking into a new life. I feel more strongly centred in the sureness of my artistic nature, able to draw and paint once more, but my concept of creativity has expanded to include healing and writing. I have had the privilege of sharing my experience with others, and the joy of facilitating a deeper, wider understanding of the infinite potential that lies within us all.

The profound shift which took place on the inner level, in the dream where I met and began to cooperate with the Inner Healer, has taken me into a new level of understanding about the nature of true healing. My feet are on a pathway which is now clearly emerging out of darkness and into the sunlight as it climbs towards the summit of the mountain. It has also brought me to the place where I am finding my true voice – able to say: I am the Healer of my Life.

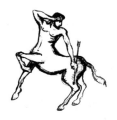

SEVEN

What are these angels who visit us
dropping through the ether in blue light
to enter our tongues,
our blood? We can only know their wisdom
and their mystery.
Remember
how the arc of their presence
is light, numinous and magical
as each day's dawn,
or stars, or birth,
or as creation, earth.

Rose Flint 1997

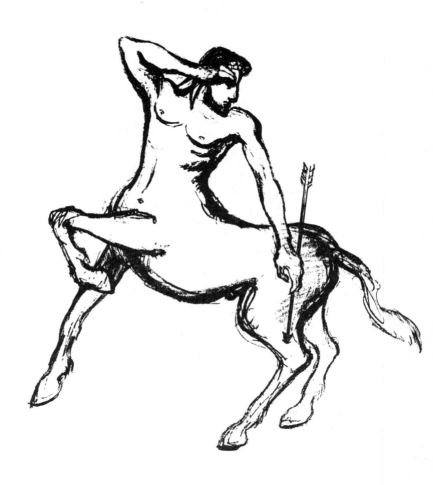

THE STORY OF CHIRON
THE WOUNDED HEALER

Mythological stories have strong archetypal themes and characters who speak universally recognised psychological truths, yet they vary in their details from one source to another. So the details of Chiron's tale will vary, not only from place to place of its telling, but, like all archetypal beings, his story is evolving and developing still as it resonates with the truth of our times.

Greek mythology, from which the story of Chiron comes, depicts the origins of our Earth and of mankind. It is a creation myth. Out of Chaos came first the mother goddess Gaia. She was the fruitful Earth. Next came Uranus, the Starry Sky with whom Gaia united, and from her womb came forth all manner of offspring, both good and evil, beneficent and monstrous. One of her sons, Cronus, castrated his father at the behest of Gaia, in revenge for having three monstrous children who she had given birth to, locked away in the earth by their father. Uranus had been so horrified by their appearance that he had hidden them away.

In these far off times when the race of man – humankind – was coming into being, great and powerful cosmic forces were at work shaping our destiny. The Hierarchy, in the form of Gods and Goddesses, Titans or Kings, Centaurs, Satyrs, and a multitude of other life-forms including the mineral, plant and animal kingdoms, were all interbreeding and interacting with one another. The power of animals was both respected and feared, and many of the ancient gods were depicted in the form of half man and half animal. The Centaurs were a race of creatures whose upper half, head and torso, was man, and the lower half was horse. They were originally employed in rounding up the bulls, the ancient counterpart perhaps, of our cowboys. But they often got rowdy and out of hand, ruled no doubt by their animal instincts, and they gave way to licentiousness and lechery.

Cronus, who had not balked at the castration of his father, the Sky God, now turned his attention to the goings-on in the world below. One fair day he came down to earth, and in a grove of trees he espied a beautiful girl, Philyra, the daughter of a king, and pursued her and tried to rape her. In panic she fled from him, and the gods, seeing her plight,

225

turned her into a mare in order to escape. He thereupon turned himself into a stallion, caught her and mated with her. She then gave birth to a boy-child with four hairy legs. Horrified and disgusted, she rejected this little monster, and abandoned him.

Deserted and disowned by both his father and his mother, the baby Chiron was found and taken to the god Apollo, who loved him and fostered him as his son. The foundling began his life deeply wounded by his mother's rejection, carrying with him always the knowledge that his lower instincts, and possibly his sexuality, had been the cause of his rejection. But he began to thrive in the warmth of the Sun God's love. Apollo was god of music, beauty, harmony, logic and reason. Under Apollo's guardianship he was educated so his higher faculties and his intellect were fostered and his creativity was developed.

In his turn, Chiron became a wise and devoted teacher, leader and healer. His instincts gave him access to knowledge of the natural world, and to the healing powers of herbs and plants. Many were the students who were drawn to him, both from the world of men and from the immortals. These included Hercules, and Apollo's favourite son, Asclepius, who was to be known as the father of medicine.

During one of the battles, which were constantly taking place between the civilised men and the savage and licentious centaurs, Hercules, who was defending the Greeks, let fly a poisoned arrow which accidentally pierced Chiron's leg. It would have been fatal but for the fact that Chiron was an immortal. Doubly wounded now, the greatest of all healers, unable to be healed and unable to die, was fated to exist in agony until the Titan, Prometheus, heard of his plight.

It was Prometheus who had created the race of man in the likeness of the gods, fashioning them from clay and water. Devoted to his creation, he stole Divine Fire from the fiery chariot of the Sun, and bestowed this gift on mankind. The race of man, however, was not yet ready to handle this intensely powerful gift. Sometimes, they were inspired to use it wisely and rose to the heights of human creation, but often, down the ages they have created chaos and destruction with the Divine Fire. The Divinities were outraged by Prometheus' theft and punished him. He was sentenced to be chained naked to a rock for the rest of his life, while a vulture tore out his liver, which grew again each day, so that his torment went on ceaselessly.

It was at this point that the two tormented souls, Prometheus and Chiron came together and evolved a creative solution. Chiron was so moved by the Titan's plight that he changed places and exchanged his immortality for the mortality of Prometheus, and died. Because of his sacrifice, the gods transformed him into a star in the heavens. Thus the immortal experienced death, the condition which all humans must pass through, until they have developed the spiritual gifts of insight, compassion, unconditional love, and have mastered the Promethean gift, divine creativity.

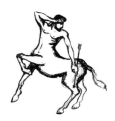

ASTRAZZURRA COMMENTS ON 'THE WOUNDED HEALER'

We wish to thank you all for participating in this journey. We do so with the sense of responsibility it has placed upon us in addressing you, and also the delight it has entailed in coming this far together. In this shared journey we have allowed a process of healing to take place. To the extent that you, the reader, have empathised with the story, you have opened a pathway within yourselves. Sunlight has filtered into areas which may have become stagnant or static, or where your creativity was stifled. In old lumber-rooms or childhood nurseries you may have discovered forgotten treasures covered in dust. Now you can take them out, dust them down and polish them up, and some of them will begin to shine and glow and give off a radiant light. It is often so. The things we repress and reject deserve better treatment. They are like the prima materia of the alchemic process. The dross falls away and the heavy metal is refined and turned to gold when we open it up to the light in this way.

In recounting her story of the sculptor's casting process (page 207) Esmé employed a metaphor which illustrated how qualities of spirit can imbue our everyday life and literally transform our earthly bodies. In symbolic terms the clay represents the ego-self, the self which identifies with the life of the body, and may be only minimally aware of its spiritual origin and power. We see how malleable clay can be impressed by outside influences during our journey from birth through our early life. Our shape is moulded by the environment, and often by our parents and teachers to fit in with their image of how they think we should be. Sadly they may think they are doing a good job if they mould us to their will. But the molecules of the clay hold the imprint of our essential being, even though others are trying to shape us.

As we get older, we take upon ourselves more and more of the shaping process. We try out first this shape and then that. Sometimes we freely choose to learn from others, at other times we resist when authority tries to impose its concepts on us. The shapes we create can be many and varied, beautiful, magnificent, weird or bizarre. But sooner or later we come to understand that the true essence within the clay is resonating to

*a higher and greater force than the one which is going about its business
of learning to create shapes or personalities.*

*However skilled we become at this self-crafting, there comes a time
when we catch the sound of the voice of a higher and greater Self (our
true note) directing us to a higher and greater purpose. This may bring
upon us a crisis of identity. We have struggled to establish our identity
through long years of testing, trials and errors. We have learned to
strengthen our ego so that it will not be subject to the ego and will of
others. This is good! This is a necessary learning objective for us. But
we may begin to see how human life can become too dominated by this
battle of the egos. Our life becomes one of struggle to gain power or to
protect power. Always we are on the watch for those who encroach and
aggress, and hope to gain advantage over us. This was one of the
strongest factors which motivated you, Esmé, to escape from London:
the competition for power which people engaged in, rather than the
more civilised urge towards cooperation.*

*In the history of your illness you were to see clearly how even those
who had dedicated themselves to the noble art of healing could be con-
taminated by this urge for power. The tyranny of the so-called 'healthy,'
over the so-called 'sick', the male ethos over the female, the strong in
authority over the weak and vulnerable, was a bid for possession of
power. You learned that there was a power struggle even in the medical
profession.*

*The ego self, at some point, begins to hear the call of the Higher Self
or true essence, and this may result in stresses. It may seem at first to the
struggling ego that its time has come. It is being called home to die. The
ego is so attached to the body-consciousness that it reacts with animal
fear when it senses the approach of its death. The unconscious intelligence of the body is programmed to survive at all costs, and senses that
those changes which it feels taking place in the body's cells as the higher
energy vibrations come in, are an attack upon its life. Unconsciously it
struggles and resists. But the clay is about to be transformed into shining golden substance. In your symbolism, a protective mould is placed
all around the clay and it is lowered into the tank or vessel where the
magical transformation will take place. Slowly the clay is withdrawn,
and there is a sense of panic at the thought of being left hollow and
empty. This can cause tension. The protective outer coating, if it is
caught up in the ego's fear, will become a tight restricting corset. It is
not yet used to the feel of the new material which is gradually pouring
in. It doesn't recognise the new self. It keeps remembering the self that
has been. That is all it knows at present.*

From the moment the magical inner healer appeared to you in your dreams, and you participated in the ritual, and accepted your role as co-creator with the Divine Essence, you experienced your connection with your Higher Self and with the Source.

You have also undertaken the role of the Wounded Healer. Those who truly heal are those who can also be in the place of the wounded and the vulnerable. The true healer comes not from the place of authority over, but authority within – becomes the author of their being. Chiron, The Wounded Healer, is a new archetype for our times. It speaks to the medical profession and patient alike. The arrow that pierces the flesh confers the gift which heals. It heals the chasm which divides those who stand on either side. Again we are confronted by the polarities. 'Health' needs 'Illness'; they are contracted to exist together. 'Victims' need 'Perpetrators' in order to play out the drama together. Whichever personality we manifest to the world is our conscious creation, and reflects our present belief system. The unmanifest is our shadow. That is the side of us we despise, reject or fear. Those we meet in life who give us the most trouble, make us feel the most uncomfortable, are often those who carry our projected shadow. If we feel inferior, we meet superiority, pride and arrogance in others. If we feel superior we may despise and mistreat the weak or vulnerable. Neither of these opposites are healing qualities. In this situation none of the players on either side of the polar drama is truly whole. True healing comes when we begin to recognise that there are echoes of the other *within us.*

The healer must learn detachment, but not the detachment which puts the sufferer at a distance, and makes the one ministering to him invulnerable from pain and distress. This continues the drama of separation. We must find a way of detachment which will protect us from being so drawn into the suffering of our patient, that we become ineffectual and subjective, yet one that allows us to be human and feeling, and even fallible. Then patients can take more responsibility for their own symptoms, realising that within the symptom lies the key to understanding the illness. Then together they can begin to make the journey towards wholeness. More healing is done through sensitive attention and clear, objective evaluation by both sides of the compact, than through all the drugs. When this level of attention is given, and the heart is open and available, then the power of healing can shine through.

ASTRAZZURRA'S MESSAGE FOR THE WORLD

Greetings to you all. I have come from afar on this occasion to be with you. If I may speak playfully in symbols I should say, many moons and stars of travel have brought me towards you to speak with you today. I have come from a distant star at a dazzling speed in light and sound. A river of light has carried me on its tidal momentum to be here with you. I am slowing now. I need to slow, so as to synchronise with my channeller, so as to be comfortable with her vibrations.

I bring you messages from far shores of the Universe. I am a traveller and I have a mission. I come to you with tidings. A tide of Light brings me to you.

These tides flow between distant shores and connect us in the same great sea. The sea of communication. The element of travel: the element by which sound is communicated. Sound which resonates within your bodies. Yes, because you are made of the same stuff as the stars, the seas, the sounds of the Universe. You are universal sound as I am, and we connect and sing together. When I speak or sound within Esmé, she carries the sound in her voice to you, and we all resonate together.

I am a blue wave of Light. A tide of the Ocean of Love which washes the Universe from end to end. All shores interconnect. All are one in harmony together.

You are my beloved children of Light. I am gathering you together in my outstretched arms and enfolding you in my heart. I come to you on wings of light and love and enter into your hearts, if you will allow me. I listen for your questionings and wonder what I can bring to you. What thoughts are forming in your minds. What you wish to ask. What messages would be most appropriate to give to you at this time.

I see something of your concerns. I see enormous trouble in your world. Great changes; transition, turbulence, and turmoil. Fear, greed and violence. Many wonder how the world they know will survive in the midst of all this chaos and upheaval. The wars, the cruelties, which engulf you at present. It is a stormy sea indeed and many are being shipwrecked in the crashing waves, and many more will be so before the storm abates.

Yet light is being created inside the dark thrashing waves. New sparks and sparkles of energising light are being created as they crash against the rocks. It is as though an 'oxygen' was being released from the vigour of the motion of chaos. An effervescence filled with fresh elements that give new energy when it is breathed in.

As it is breathed in you will take it into yourselves – into your blood and build new cells. The whole body will be renewed, and by this I mean the whole body of humankind. The old body of mankind is disintegrating, and you need to let it go. There is no point at all in hanging on to the ageing corpse in the hope that it will be resurrected. There are some who look to technology and a new science of cryonics to preserve the body in the hope that this will preserve life. There can be no new life until we pass through death. Preserving the worn out outer casing of the soul in the hope that new life can be grafted onto it in the form of spare parts, or that immortality can be injected into it in some future way, is a rather horrible mistake.

The mortal body which we own at present must decay and go to earth or to fire, then it will release to us, as we depart, essences which will spiritualise and be incorporated into our spiritual bodies. If we attempt to preserve the corpse we interrupt the process and hinder our flowering into the spiritual body. We will be captured and held down by this strange technological intervention. Weighted down and chained to earth by our fear when we need to fly freely and expand into our light bodies.

You need to face death and go through it, and not get side-tracked by techniques by which you hope to avoid this transition, for this will prevent your understanding of the incredible process of release which death brings. The possibilities awaiting you are immense. Your own creativity and imagination can be harnessed in the formation of your new being.

Humanity will go through a transition stage at the point where you are now. Most will inevitably die, but it can be a wonderful experience. Let go your fear and open your arms to it. As your fear recedes, so the diseases which plague you at present will recede also. Death need not be a process of pain, degeneration and waste. Embrace it and it will respond to you and you can let your body drop from you as a leaf from a tree in the autumn sunshine.

Each day you can die a little this way, and each day you will breathe in new life. Every time you allow yourself to lightly shed a leaf, your living body changes. It becomes lighter and also stronger. It takes into itself more of the vibration of light and also more of the substance of earth until it becomes a living fountain; an exchange process. Drinking in through its roots the sustaining life force of the planet Earth from which it builds its cellular structure, and breathing in the new elemental oxygen from the air. It will be a constant fountain of renewal.

Those who learn to embrace death learn the secret of life, and they will also see how they can heal the planet which mankind has ravaged. Embrace the destruction and chaos which will come, by being rooted in the earth and centred within your Heart Centre in the holy love which flows in on the universal tide. Let it sing through you and play upon you like a harp, singing its melody outwards, and thus you will play your part in the composition of the New Earth Symphony.

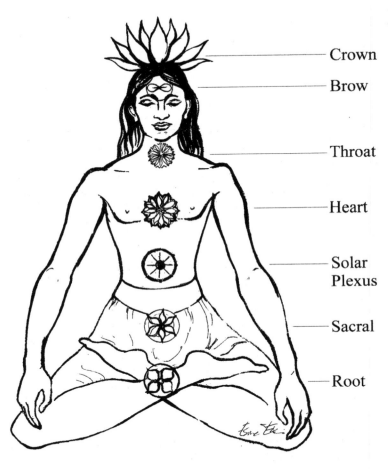

Crown

Brow

Throat

Heart

Solar
Plexus

Sacral

Root

The Seven Major Chakras
See Appendix for a description of the Chakra System

A GUIDED MEDITATION

FOR ROOTING, HEALING AND TRANSFORMING
THE PHYSICAL BODY

For this meditation, seat yourself comfortably, either on a chair with your spine upright and your back supported, or in the Lotus position. Relax, close your eyes, and breathe naturally and rhythmically, letting your hands rest in your lap. As you breathe, let your focus be in your Heart Chakra, which is on a level with your physical heart, and begin to breath in and out from there.

With the breath-energy leading you, allow yourself to travel in your imagination to a beautiful landscape, a green meadowland nourished by water ... Wander at will among the wild flowers, touching the delicate petals, smelling the fragrances, listening to the sounds. Pausing by herbs, plants or trees, where you can taste whatever taste experiences are offered to you ... It is a place of freshness, and newness, everything awakening to new life and growth. Although it might seem familiar at first, soon, as you breathe in the fresh air, even the familiar becomes transformed. The greenness is more vibrant, intense, more real, more alive than anywhere you have been or experienced before.

As you breathe in the air you are aware of a wonderful light ... Through your breath you will begin to draw down the Spiritual Light so that it infuses the earth, and infuses your physical body ... A golden sun above you smiles down and you feel its warmth entering your being. It has a healing quality and radiance ... As you breathe in, let this radiance enter the Crown petals. At the top of your head are the petals of the Crown Chakra. They are of the finest white substance; translucent, iridescent, and reflecting in the atoms of their structure, every colour in the spectrum, but the colour which is most present, especially at their base where they come to meet your head, is translucent violet.

As these delicate petals begin to open, they may remind you of the forms of water lilies or lotus flowers. As the light warms them and they open out, it is as though a beautiful flower was emerging out of a serene pool of clear blue etheric water. The flower has a stalk which goes down to the bed of the pool. To the fertile mud at the bottom where the root is situated ... You are as serene as the still, clear pool, and the flexible stalk goes down through the centre of your body following your spine. At its top it bears the wondrous flower which draws in the light and the air from above. This then travels down the stalk, through your body as you breathe in, and as you breathe out it continues down the stalk to its root in the bed of the pool, and is breathed out down into the earth.

Pause

Feel the breath and feel *your* roots going down into the earth ... With the next breath draw into your roots the life-giving energy of the earth. It rises up the stalk effortlessly, and flows out into the light above the petals of your Crown Flower ... As you continue to breathe in this way, you become aware of your body and your whole spiritual being coming into alignment, as the light-filled stalk balances your Crown Flower at its tip, anchored securely by the root system, which is fed and held by the earth. Your Root Chakra is at the base of your spine between your legs and points downwards.

Pause

Just allow yourself to grow and to flow and to flourish as this green stalk of Light and Life supports you.

Pause

As you continue to breathe in this way, be aware of the other five centres situated on the central column or stalk filling with the appropriate light and colour as the breath descends. Situated at intervals on this stalk are the other major chakra centres of your body. Just below the Crown Flower is the Brow centre, like a rich, deep blue flower between and just above the eyes, with its petals opening out to the front and its stem behind the head ... Feel the breath flowing through and filling the centre of the indigo flower as it descends. It then comes into the flower of the Throat chakra, filling it with translucent sky blue light ... Your breath continues downwards through the stalk to your Heart level, where it enters the centre of the Heart Flower. Here you sense a vibrant soft green light filling the petals of this flower, which open out also to the front of your body with its counterpoint at the back between the shoulder blades ... Your breath travels downwards and into the centre of the Solar Flower in your solar plexus and it is filled with clear sunshine yellow ... Your breath descends as you breathe and comes down into the abdomen. Here it fills the Sacral Flower, which is just below the navel, with amber orange light.

Gradually let your focus come into your Root Chakra. Its petals face down towards the earth and they glow with a rosy red light. Imagine that you also have a strong tap root which goes deep into the earth. Follow the urge of the life force within the root, and feel your feet sinking into the moist, brown, fertile earth. The whole of your physical body now feels nourished and revitalised by the earth. An energy exchange is taking place. Your body is releasing its tensions, its fatigue, its pain. You feel able to release into the earth old negative emotions which your body has stored. You feel the time has come to let them go ... You are experiencing an exchange contract with the earth. All that is now ready to be released from your body – residues of outworn experiences which you have held on to, past resentments, distress. Or there may be things which have gone deeper still to fester and cause dis-ease. Through the angelic power of transmutation they become fertiliser for new growth and regeneration.

A process takes place in the earth as the dark, heavy substances are released. Through your stalk connection with the light of the Spiritual Sun, the planet can receive the energy she needs for her own transformation. The element which surrounds and carries the plant is the etheric body. The etheric lake supports the plant, the body physical. It is a blue lake which washes away the exuded substances as they are released from the body, and carries them away to mingle with the earth at the bottom of the lake.

Pause

Green leaves are forming on the stalk and spreading out into the physical body. These are the lungs of the plant. They breathe the energy of the Heart Chakra, the green chlorophyll of the plant, synthesised from the sunlight and air that comes in at the Crown ... Feel these green leaves sprouting right through your body transmitting light into your cells. Regenerating your blood, your bones, your tissues ... The plant of your being has rooted in the earth. Let it grow and breathe, expanding throughout your body until every cell is clean and sparkling with light.

Stay with this feeling as long as you wish and are comfortable. Then gradually return to everyday consciousness. Become aware of your physical breath in your physical body. Feel your feet firmly on the ground, and open your eyes. Orientate yourself with your surroundings, and before you resume your occupations, close each chakra and protect it with a cross of light within a circle of light, and draw a cloak of white light all around you, above your head and below your feet.

OBSERVATION ON THE TWO FIGURES
'YOUTH' AND 'THE WINGED MAN'

Around the time A.Z. was dictating the Eighth Commentary, he inti-
mated that there was something more he would like to say about our
creations. I became aware as I recollected that period when I lived in
Rome, that even though the two sculptures, Youth and The Winged Man,
were no longer physically existing, their 'presence' was still active. A.Z.
tells us that everything that is put out, word or deed, has a continuing
resonance which affects the present. Collectively, our positive or negative creations become records in the ether; personally, they are energy
forces within our psyche, which can be accessed and made conscious.
With that, further creative possibilities open up. We can consciously
choose to review the past, dissolve and let go those things which no
longer serve us, but also in alignment with our spiritual dimension, we
can integrate dynamic qualities which have become lost to us. This empowers us by allowing us to take our life into our own hands,
transforming it and healing it.

The following observations from A.Z. were taken from a wealth of information he dictated, and from which he asked me to select what I felt
would be useful for the readers. The visualisation, or guided journey, in
'Mystical Marriage' which concludes the book, illustrates beautifully the
powerful transformative effect which flows from this kind of creative
work.

I asked him if he could remind us first of the birth vision which he had
spoken about in his First Commentary.

*Before birth, in the between-life state, we receive a clearer picture of
our previous lives and gain an understanding of the human impulses and
conditions which entrapped us and diverted us from our intentions. We
set out with a plan, we chose our place of birth and our immediate relations in the life to come, in order to bring us the optimum experiences
for development. For learning lessons which would clear us from negative bonds which tied us to lower states of consciousness shrouded in
darkness, illusion and ignorance. In the between-life state, much work is
done to free ourselves from the darkness which blinkered us while on*

Earth. We experience again the wonderful exhilaration of this freedom, and vow never again to become trapped. So we set off with high hopes. Our teachers in the higher dimensions will have given us much help by feeding us with the combined insights and love energy of the Soul Group, and it will be a clear choice that we have made, to strive while on Earth to realise that wonderful freedom and vision once again.

[That which inspires and animates us can, if not recognised and acted upon positively, also become repressed. It lives a life of its own in the unconscious.]

The two sculptures which played such an important part for Esmé at the time she was in Rome, carried the energy of inspiration. Inspiration, like our most creative dreams, comes to us from the spiritual dimensions. It flows from our Divine Vision, fanned by the Breath which animated us at our conception when our spark leapt free from the mind of God and began to travel outwards down the ages, expanding into consciousness. We who have travelled a little further on, only long to add our breath to that wind so that your flame can grow and glow more brightly. In striving to bring to perfection one's visions, we may lose sight of the impulse which fired them and they may sink back into the darkness of the womb, waiting to try again. They become lost aspects of our greater personality and lie beneath the surface like other relegated parts of our self, subpersonalities, needing us to love them and recognise them and own them. Then they can ascend and transform and perhaps come into their full power.

As you have observed Esmé, 'Youth' was for you a seminal piece: a signpost if you like, pointing to the future. The original figure did, in fact, have its right arm extended outwards as if pointing ahead. You spoke of its energy as being 'Spring', an uncoiling force spiralling out from the centre. It expresses well the creative well-spring which is the source of your true essence.

He who began as an inspired idea, before becoming translated into artistically expressed form, carried an energy whose intention was to communicate feeling. Because you became ashamed of his artistic shortcomings, somewhere along the way he got lost, and his energy sank back into the womb of creation from which it had emerged. But such was the force of the energy that it found ways to express itself unconsciously. He, or the creative force he carried, had the power to shape matter, and constructed a wall of defence from your body's material. We all begin to create these character armours as we emerge from childhood to protect the beautiful but sensitive original self we

239

were at birth, and our creativity is diverted into such pathways as survival strategies.

We are all born with creative potential, since we are sparks from the Divine Creative Source. Yet many of us do not, or dare not realise it. The creative impulse, because it is Love, draws together. As Esmé began to grow up and assume the mantle of creative artist, it drew together the threads of her innate love of stone and rock as carved by natural forces of wind and rain, or stressed, pressured and metamorphosed by heat and cold. It drew secret and tender passions of youth, as well as its dynamic active energy. A sculptor or an architect comes into life with a mission and a vocation clearly imprinted. They have a vision to realise. A vision so strong, that they are drawn to Earth by a force of love for the body of the planet. The very particles of Earth move, dance and respond to the music which the artist's soul is playing, and he or she communes, albeit unconsciously, with nature and the spirits of nature in the form of the Angelic and Devic kingdoms. The true artist communes with vast universal archetypal forces of Harmony, Beauty and Sacred Geometry and offers him/herself as an instrument for the transmission of that Soul Music. We work with the Beautiful Ones to solidify and crystallise universal sound, and we structure these lyrics and symphonies into visible and tangible shapes and spaces on Earth. Morphic resonance.

[How the impulse to express in outer form went inward.]

But the resonance of Youth, this sculptural work, was thwarted and frustrated when it couldn't find satisfactory expression in outward form. The only outlet for it eventually was to create a stronger defensive fortress, inside whose walls beat a loving, living heart. So the defences grew and the heart repined – while communication was lost. It surfaced again in the vision of a Winged Man. Once more, a tender creature inspired by the bird, inside a powerful structure. Only this time it was the structure of wings. So you initiated in the same year, these two figures. One expressing Earth's weight and her slow aeons of growth, the other immediate, soaring, almost weightless. Earth-bound and Heaven bound. Opposites in these two extremes, yet in their vulnerability they were similar.

You had a strong mental image of a male creative energy inside you. This is very much like your inner male counterpoint or animus, that inner being which animates and inspires the female – just as the anima does for man. For you at that period he embodied your creative male strength, that which you needed as a sculptress (let's call you by the feminine form) to carry out the 'work', the alchemic work, the work of creation. Your artistic intent was to capture, within his human form, some of the elements and textures of the great stone faces and edges of the landscape of your youth, which you had been intimately 'in touch' with. The mountains of North Wales and the Derbyshire edges of mill-stone grit which had been carved out of the landscape by the slow, determined action of the elements. You wished to juxtapose the ancient, long enduring hardness of the mineral kingdoms with the fleeting, thrilling tenderness of springtime, all in one figure. This expressed something of your own true spirit.

Yet there was something more expressing itself. Something in the womb of unconsciousness which you didn't recognise at all. You were also drawing forth from yourself in his rock-like exterior, a bulwark against the tides of life which you sensed were inundating you. Inside himself he was tender as a spring leaf unfurling. He had love in his heart. Longing for tenderness to be met by love. He was sensitive flesh and blood which was vulnerable to being hacked to pieces by sharp, destructive criticism and by judgements from on high. So he built an armour so strong that his male energy became consolidated in a strength which immobilised his feelings. This became your inner unconscious negative creation which grew in strength and became immensely powerful, a 'Colossus' in fact. You may question now if it has served you well, or has it become too strong, and is it time to let it go and allow the true creative seed within the heart to blossom in gentle power?

[The consciousness/energy of the Heart Chakra as it develops, brings us 'in touch with' … In esoteric terms it is the Feeling Body through which we relate directly, tenderly, empathetically, without defences or barriers, to people, to nature and to the universe.]

Can we look at the energy centre we call the Heart Chakra for a moment? The heart is a bridge connecting our spiritual being with our earthly being. The main colour this chakra radiates is spring green. The sense associated with it is touch, and its expression is feeling. Feeling as distinct from emotion, which is the expression of the Sacral Chakra – two stops below.

Centred in the Heart we can breathe up from the chakras immediately below, the energy/consciousness from the Sacral (emotion) and the clear energy (rational thought) from the Solar Plexus, and balance these functions so that a new level of feeling is created. No longer is there the duality, thought vs. emotion, but thoughtfulness tempering raw emotion, and the fluidity of feeling softening and deepening thought. In the Heart, new qualities of evaluation, compassion, wisdom, love detached from subjective over-involvement, can open up, allowing us to develop a more honest relationship with other people and the natural world. Awakening the Heart allows synthesis and balance. In the Heart Centre we learn to be open hearted but not too open that we ignore our own needs. We realise our first duty is to our own health and well-being, so that we preserve a source within us that we can share with others. We realise our connection to nature and to the Universal source of life-energy which fills us with love.

Our Earth is evolving and changing, as we who live on her and feed from her are changing. We are what we eat. We sustain our lives from mother Earth, and the mineral kingdom is in our cells and our bones and blood. We fortify ourselves physically and build up fortresses in our psyche from the psychic energy of earth. We are indistinguishable from our planet. We are created out of her body and our consciousness resonates with her consciousness. Our aura mingles with her aura.

Yet at the same time we are at war with ourselves, with one another, and with our planet! That mystical, harmonious oneness which we shared with all creation as we began our long journey down the evolutionary chain to emerge as primitive man, and which we still retained at that early stage, became gradually lost as we gained greater consciousness.

[The new-born infant stage of evolution.]

The gift of consciousness and free will, which we earned for ourselves, has taken us further away from that original harmonious unity which was ours, yet was ours unconsciously. Consciousness has brought us to a point of split, severing the basic unity asunder. It placed an awesome god-like power in our hands. We have divided dark from light, created 'good' and 'evil' and choice. We on this planet stand out in dangerous, splendid isolation from the whole of creation. If we choose to retrieve the situation; if we choose to relate, to love, to unite, to heal the split within us, we will go on to create a world which is unique within the Universe. Ours is a planet of conscious choice and of healing. A great cosmic experiment will have come to pass. A new Heaven and a new Earth will be born and the whole universe will sing.

But we have a situation of great danger before us. How will we choose? Will you choose healing or self-destruction? There is no other option. If healing is chosen it implies a leap in consciousness out of the old model, which sees material existence as the only fact, and the brain as creator/producer of consciousness, into a new understanding of consciousness as the creative power which forms matter. The old mode of thinking cannot give us this understanding – so what will? It will emerge for us as we learn to raise our vibrations – our consciousness levels – into the Heart chakra and from there lift up and link with the three higher chakras. The Throat, the Brow and the Crown.

* * *

My message has always been, 'I can help you access the Higher Knowledge and the Greater Vision, but I can't carry it out for you. It is your unique vision.' This vision was available to you – to all of you – before birth. It is the vision of why we came here and what we meant to do with our earthly life. We all come 'trailing clouds of glory' then life, with its doubts and fears, intervenes. Then we die and we realise again, with horror, that we have made a mess of our once clear intentions. And once again we are given another chance. Little by little we learn, and every piece of learning hewn from the rock of our forgetting, is a jewel of light.

For so many, the window between Heaven and Earth closes soon after we are born. Bereft of that connection with spirit some grasp hold of the religious rules of their particular group to guide them, while others develop a more rational and scientific view and pour the energy of their vision into creating their Heaven on Earth, declaring 'God is dead'. It is time for a new realisation. Gradually, humanity is being drawn into a resonance, a new planetary awareness. So as we approach the conclusion of this book the message is of synthesis. My wings have descended into your earthly life: you have fashioned out of earth a vehicle to receive those wings, and in combination, matter and energy, earth and spirit rise upwards until you will find it possible to move at ease between the two planes – in and out of the material and spiritual dimensions.

Eventually there will be no need for death to occur before you can reconnect with your vision. Your physical eyes and your spiritual eyes will fuse. The Spiritual Eye will have opened at the brow level and you will literally Fly. Your struggles will be at an end. Your defences will melt away. Let your hearts sing in this knowledge. Rejoice.

SHARING THE HARVEST SUPPER

We are coming to the end of this journey. We have taken this path to-gether, climbing the mountain, reaching the peak. One person stands at the peak, yet in that one person all are present. You, the reader, stand . there, and you have brought the gift of who you are, the hidden as well as the part of you that you make present. In this journey we have shared one another. My words are an offering from the harvest of my days, a repast which I have shared with you, and my words have mingled with those of Esmé. Her harvest has also been brought to you, both the bitter fruits and the sweetness, and if you have taken in those words and di-gested them, they have become part of you. What we eat we become. We have all brought our gifts to the table and shared a communion or com-munal meal. Communion, and communication, are energy. We share one another's energy and thus we become healed. Because to be separate is to be sick. Separation is an illusion we have created as we have gone through life. When we came to this Earth, we didn't know separation at first, but we very soon forgot that we were a part of the Divine whole-ness.

So we stand at this peak and we have each brought with us a crowd, a myriad of possibilities. Many facets of our self which lie inside us still waiting for us to give them birth. We are now all learning how to fly. Each one, as the new day breaks, will take her path into the sunrise and soar into the blue: ascend to the summit of Heaven. Once you have found your wings there will be no end to your creative powers and pos-sibilities. You will go to the far shores of the Universe unlimited by time or matter, and you will carry with you the harvest you have gathered from your many lifetimes spent on Earth. What a glorious harvest to share with other beings and other lifestreams in the Universe.

The seeds of the harvest you will plant and tend, and it will spring forth into blossoms and fruits. Everywhere you go seeds will be scat-tered and blessed. A great seeding and a great harvest will take place across the skies and every planet and star will rejoice and sing. This is a great vision and a great expanding.

Yet planet Earth you will still hold dear. It is your home and its future needs to be guarded and stewarded. Much will need to be done in the coming years. The next few years will be crucial. The great momentum of negative force which has gathered over the years of historical time is rolling up and growing denser. Dark, heavy particles are congregating together as the light expands.

The great sleep in which so many lie at present will need to be broken into. Humanity's slumber, the soporific state which we have sought for ourselves, the drugged world of unreality we have escaped into to shut out fear, needs some fresh air introduced into it. Those who learn to fly will find themselves lifted into a clearer, sonant layer of atmosphere. It is from this clarity that they will begin to beam down insights that will travel into the consciousness of their fellow men and women. As each newly awakened flier lifts off, they will raise the collective level of consciousness. Soon, to a point where the thick particles which have clogged the eyes and ears of humanity, will begin to dissolve. Expect a new renaissance of science and art. Healing and creativity will go hand in hand. Environmental healers and warriors for peace, parents who can be mother/father to the child of delight.

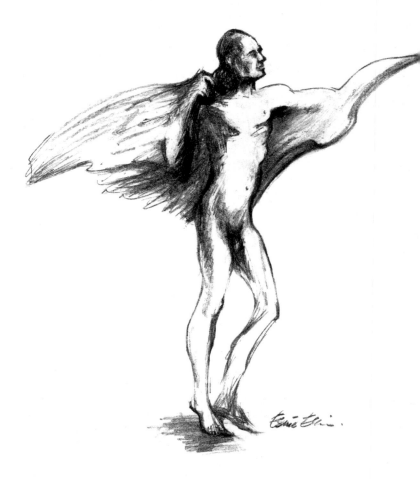

The Winged Man
Working drawing for sculpture

MYSTICAL MARRIAGE

Bringing our creative potential into consciousness and raising it. The following passage develops into what I would describe as a guided meditation with dialogue. We offer it as an illustration of how psychological and spiritual dynamics combine. The potential of Inner Personalities can be liberated, and their positive qualities integrated through the power of imagination, using visualisation and intent. Symbols used in this way can bring about substantial changes in consciousness and at the physical level. (This is not intended as an exercise. For further reading on how to structure exercises, see the Bibliography.)

Our search for spiritual meaning and purpose can be said to reflect the ascension through the chakras. With the Root Chakra representing our sense of connection with our place of birth and the Earth planet, through our developing sense of self and relationship with others at the mid level, there comes a gradual awareness of the higher Chakras. As we approach the Crown, the Top of the Mountain, a dialogue opens up with our higher wisdom and the spiritual dimensions.

In rediscovering and re-membering your relationship with those two personalities (your sculptures) who inspired you long ago, you have the opportunity of bringing two different aspects of their male energy together. With you as the third and central feminine point, a 'triadic marriage' can take place.

This place we now occupy close to the summit of the mountain, is a sacred and magical place. It has been reached by means of the long journey which started with the rooting and earthing which took place at birth. If you look down now at the scene in the valley below, you may see the path you have climbed which brought you to the mountain, and re-member the stages of growth and the places you have passed through in your life. Remembering, too, the place where you met your Inner Healer. As you pause here you become aware that Youth and The Winged Man have joined you, and there is an implicit understanding between you that a long awaited moment has come. Your greeting of one another is warm and passionate. It feels appropriate that there should be a special cere-mony at this point to honour your reunion, so the choice of the wise

247

Inner Healer to preside at the marriage would seem a happy one, since he comes from synthesis at the Heart Centre.

At this place on the mountain path where you have paused, there is a spring of clear thirst-quenching water, and warm air wafts up from the valley below carrying scents of the green wooded slopes. A massive wall of rock glinting with sunlight stands to one side of the path. A tree rooted in the rock face hides a fissure, but as you approach you see it is the entrance to a cave. Let the Inner healer lead you together into its sacred space, so that you may prepare by becoming still and settled into your deep inner centre.

It seems dark at first, but warm and dry, and there is a sense of welcoming security and deep peace. You feel your feet upon a sandy pathway which goes deeper into the cave. You follow the Healer and find yourselves entering another cave. This time it is lit by a gentle, shimmering light which seems to be radiating from all directions. As you adjust to its light you see a myriad of translucent stalactites all emitting soft ethereal colours. It is a crystal cave and the walls, ceiling and floor shimmer like rainbows; quite unearthly in their iridescent beauty. You find a place where the crystals on the floor are like fine sand, soft and silky. Here you may sit down. Breathing from your heart centre you become very still and drawn into meditation. So silent, so still, there is a dark, velvety black peace inside you. No image, no breeze ruffles the surface of your deep inner lake.

Gradually you become aware that a quiet symphony of sound is emanating from the stalactites hanging from the roof, and as you emerge from the depths of your silence, but still centred into yourselves and relaxed, the sound changes to colour. Each note becomes a different colour tone. You are bathed in a spectrum of healing colours. In a while you begin to feel energised and wide awake, and ready to move outwards again into the mountain air and the sunlight. The Healer escorts you to the cave mouth, but waits in the shade while you step outside once more.

Taking stock again of your surroundings, looking at the view. You have ascended the mountain with Youth and the Winged Man, and together joined in this wonderful meditation of healing and reunion. You have paused at this place near the summit to look back. Take a moment now to really experience in your heart the essence of your two companions. How are you now regarding your two lovers? What are your feelings now for them? In what way have they changed, and how have you changed in the way you relate to them?

I am astonished at their beauty and their strength. I appreciate in a way I never did before, their many and different qualities. The Winged Man almost on tiptoe as he reaches up like a great bird, and Youth with his feet planted firmly on the earth. In some ways I am in awe of them both, and feel I have much to learn from them. I love Youth's tenderness blended with a wild and wanton passion. His warm, muscular body has a faint animal musk and is redolent of balmy woodland scents. I guess he is rather shy, but I love his curiosity about the world and his generosity to people. If I found his connection to the eternally long, slow movement of the mineral kingdoms constricting at first, I now see more of its wisdom and patience. Youth is Eternal. He is also Potential. In his seed is potency, and this is one of the gifts he brings.

He embodies the potential for connecting with the healing medicine of plants, trees and animals: for understanding 'medicine' in its wider sense of that which intuitively unlocks the hidden knowledge, which every life-form uniquely contains, and allows the healing which flows from that reconnection to our ancient memories to be actualised.

I respect him for his caring for the environment, for his skills and craftsmanship, his understanding of the nature of materials. The grain of wood, the temperament and tensile strength of metal, the textures and character of stone. I love his innate knowledge of the seasons and animal lore. He has brought me a dream of the Turtle, which will teach me the magic of the protective shield which she is able to fashion from the wisdom of the Earth. His gift to me is Earth wisdom, but the lessons I shall learn from him as our relationship unfolds are endless.

The Winged Man carries me up in his arms. He inspires, he thrills and enraptures. His wings promise expansion and discovery. He will take me to new lands, new seas, visiting new horizons, attaining new dimensions. He will teach me new depths and heights of sound and music, he will awaken me to new colours and forms of expression. His body is warm and strong but light, and his aerial seed also is dynamic with potential. His wings reach towards the sun and extend beyond, to the furthest reaches of imagination.

Stand with one lover on either hand and you in the centre. They are beginning to attain archetypal status. One commands the Earthly powers and sings his song to which the mountains respond and the leaves dance. The other stands on tiptoe, wings outstretched and commands the Thunder and the Lightening. But for all their power there is a gentleness within them. Their love surrounds you. Let yourself be embraced by this synergy of mutual love. In love you are united and balanced. That love energy becomes a column of flowing light inside you uniting Heaven and

Earth. That hard defence which once restricted and isolated you, becomes a flowing column which supports you from within, a golden fountain which expands and fills your body. Male energy uniting with female, Yin with Yang. The gift which the feminine principle brings to the marriage is receptivity. The male energy is active. It 'carries out' in the world, it acts, but what is carried out must be carried back and be received. The feminine absorbes and contains the light, processing it within the dark vessel in which gestation takes place.

As you stand together, there forms an image of an oak tree. Its trunk draws its great strength from the granite earth, and it is decked with wild green leaves dancing in the sunlight. Its great tap root throbs with the pulse of the life within the earth, while above its crown thunder rolls and lightning splays dazzling diamond spears. The gods pay homage to its wisdom and age.

The tree remembers, for its past and future are timelessly present. It remembers being struck by the awesome power of the lightning, its trunk split asunder and the fire penetrating it and consuming its heart wood. It burnt in a violent intense heat until it was left blackened and hollow. One might expect it now to be doomed, but it is not so. Such are its powers of regeneration that, as the seasons pass, new roots grow into the earth and begin to feed and draw up the sap which filters through to the tissues and cells of the outer layers of the old tree. New branches grow, new leaves are put out. Safe in a crook of one of those branches is a nest, and in that nest is a warm egg. Inside that egg is a yolk of golden fire.

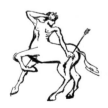

AFTERWORD

As people begin to search and ask real, existential questions, 'Why am I here?' 'What is my purpose in life?' or when they signal in some way that they are ready for guidance or healing at a deeper level, there comes a growing awareness of synchronicity – timing of events. Then meaningful coincidences, the right person, phone call or book may appear at the right moment. The fact of this book being in your hands at this moment may be one sign that you are receptive to such communication. This may lead you to the next book which will answer further questions, or the unexpected, but right journey may materialise, and that will lead you on. Your journey has begun.

Esmé Ellis 1998

BIBLIOGRAPHY

Ruth White & Mary Swainson, *Gildas Communicates*, C.W. Daniel & Co. Ltd

Ruth White, *A Question Of Guidance**, C.W.Daniel & Co. Ltd

    *Working With Your Chakras**, Piatkus Books

    *Working With Guides And Angels**, Piatkus Books

    *The River Of Life**, Piatkus

Barbara Ann Brennan, *Hands Of Light**, Bantam Books

    *Light Emerging**, Bantam Books

Deepak Chopra, *Quantum Healing*, Bantam Books

James Redfield, *The Celestine Prophesy*, Warner Books

    The Tenth Insight, Bantam Books

Marlo Morgan, *Mutant Message From Down-Under*, Thorsons

Piero Ferrucci, *What We May Be**, Thorsons

* Books giving specific exercises/guided meditations.

APPENDIX

THE CHAKRA SYSTEM

In illustrations of Hindu Yoga meditation, we often see wheels of light depicting chakras down the centre front of the body, and sited at major subtle energy centres. We live surrounded by invisible energies: around us personally is an energy field known in esoteric terms as an aura, and this has seven layers, each one finer and subtler than the next. The densest closest to the physical body.

These energies not only surround but interpenetrate the physical body, and chakras can be thought of as gateways through which they flow. Like the musical scale, as they ascend from the base of the body towards the top, they emit a tonal vibration, which can be observed by trained psychic vision, or Higher Sense Perception, as colours. The slowest vibration is at the Root Chakra, which is at the base of the body between the legs. Its main colour is red. The fastest vibration is at the Crown Chakra at the top of the head and its colour is violet. There are seven major chakras, though higher spiritual sources are now indicating others, rather like new planets being discovered. But for simplicity's sake I shall describe only seven.

Each of these chakras is a little world of consciousness reflecting a stage in our growth and evolution. Any disease or psychological disturbance will show up here. In complete health all are in alignment and their colours clear, vibrant and their textures flexible. What these chakras reveal is that we have within us the potential for full realisation of our essential being. They represent, if you like, a journey of healing (wholeness) and learning (wisdom).

The Root Chakra is mainly red. It reflects the consciousness of the infant: its birthing and its earthing experience during the first three years of life. If all has gone well and we have been nurtured with love and security as well as the right nourishment, healthy foundations will have been established and the chakra will glow in response. It responds to the Earth element and grounds us into physical life.

255

The Sacral Chakra is mainly orange. The stage of consciousness here is from the age of three to eight. Important emotional development is taking place, and an awareness of gender. Creativity and empowerment are closely linked with the energy of developing sexuality. If the earlier stage of nurturing has been neither too harsh nor too free, relationships with other people and with the outer world will follow successfully. There is a link here to the element of Water.

The Solar Plexus Chakra is mainly yellow. As its name suggests it is a sun centre and also a complex centre. The warm, clear, yellow energy provides the evolutionary impetus for the development of intellectual powers. Reason, Logic, Opinion. Around this stage, eight to twelve years, a strong sense of self is developing. The ego consciousness comes to the fore. Here the element is Fire.

The Heart Chakra is mainly green. The developmental stage is twelve to fifteen. The emotions which began to be generated in the Sacral area, and which might often have been fierce and overwhelming forces, begin to be consciously recognised by the developing thought processes at the Solar Plexus stage. In the Heart Chakra a new level of feeling is reached. The green energy and the vibrational level here, bring us in touch with people and nature through a sense of love and relatedness. Thought and feeling come together (Wisdom). Sexual love at the level of tenderness and ecstasy is felt. At-oneness with life, nature, and with the 'other': a state beyond ego-consciousness. The element here is Air.

The Throat Chakra is mainly (sky) blue. Developmental age is fifteen to twenty-one. We 'come of age'. These three last chakras are the highest spiritual centres with the Throat being a bridge between the levels. Its energy is of expression and communication, and where this centre is spiritually awakened it expands communication into a realisation of our Truth. We discover Vocation. The element is Ether.

The Brow Chakra is mainly Indigo. It is beyond a developmental age. Its Sanskrit name is 'Ajna' meaning 'command'. The Brow brings vision of our true purpose, inspiration and communion with the Higher Mind, and the command of our Spirit.

The Crown Chakra is mainly Violet. It is the Temple at the top of the mountain where we may meet our Higher Self, and connect once again with our soul group and are reminded of our original life's intent or birth vision. The struggling, stubborn ego relaxes and dissolves as we flow and blend harmoniously with our Higher Will. New strength is available when this chakra opens to the Divine Source.